Reflections

ON BEING A PHYSICIAN

Reflections

ON BEING A PHYSICIAN

ROBERT G. HOOPER M.D.

JUST PEACHY PRESS

For information, please contact Just Peachy Press, P.O. Box 4100 Scottsdale, AZ 85261-4100; fax: 480-998-3622 or email justpeachypress@att.net.

Editorial assistance: Leta Waugh at Scribendi
Cover and interior design: Jennifer Stimson
Cover photo Bust of Hippocrates: PhilSigin
First printing: 2025

Names: Hooper, Robert G., author.
Title: Reflections on being a physician / Robert G. Hooper, M.D.
Description: Includes bibliographical references. | Scottsdale, AZ: Just Peachy Press, 2025.
Identifiers: LCCN: 2025913686 | ISBN: 979-8-9893631-2-4 (paperback) | 979-8-9893631-3-1 (ebook)
Subjects: LCSH Hooper, Robert G. | Physicians--Biography. | Medicine. | Medicine--Biography. | Physician-Patient Relations. | Medical ethics. | Essays. | BISAC BIOGRAPHY & AUTOBIOGRAPHY / Memoirs | BIOGRAPHY & AUTOBIOGRAPHY / Medical | MEDICAL / Essays | MEDICAL / Ethics | MEDICAL / Physicians and Patients
Classification: LCC R153 .H66 2025 | DDC 610.92--dc23

For Dana

Table of Contents

Prologue xi

Acknowledgements xiii

Essays on the Practice of Medicine

SECTION ONE

Learning The Ropes – Introduction To Section One 17

The Best Doctor In The World 20

Acts Of God Or Acts Of Man 25

Links In A Chain 30

Responsibilities 34

Attitude 38

Success 42

Tools 46

The Telephone Call 50

Mrs. B And The Art Of Medicine 52

The Picard Syndrome 56

Quiet Please 59

The Ride 63

Essays on The American Medical System

SECTION TWO

Medicine as a Business – Introduction to Section Two...69
How Are You Paid?...72
The Make a Car Program...76
"A Right To Healthcare" – It Is Not That Simple...79
A Line in the Sand...83
Boards...87
"Open the Pod Bay Doors, Hal"
Or, A Tool Doctors Should Control...91
Titles...96
The Business of Medicine...100

Defining a Physician

SECTION THREE

Defining a Physician –Introduction to Section Three...109
A Doctor? No, a Physician...113
A Doctor's Oath...122
The Hippocratic Oath...129
Physicians, Doctors and The Oath...138
Healthcare Workers, Providers, Doctors and
Physicians...143
Medical Societies, Associations and Colleges...149
Who, then, Is a Physician?...155

Epilogue and a Calling

SECTION FOUR

Epilogue and a Calling 165

A Classical Hippocratic Oath 2025 167

Nightingale Pledge* 169

Physician Assistant Oath 170

Final Thioughts.. 171

Bibliography.. 173

Prologue

Being recognized as a Physician[1] is the highest honor a Doctor of Medicine[2] can achieve. Any Doctor of Medicine can be one. Few are. Far fewer are recognized as one. It is a quest of a lifetime.

Being a Physician is about character, civility, responsibility, questioning, self-reflection, and personal honor. It is not about training, medical or surgical specialty, experience, expertise, or employment. This book is about what distinguishes a Physician from a Doctor of Medicine.

All writing has some purpose, be it to express an opinion, relieve the author's frustrations, change mankind, or just boost an ego. This volume likely exists for all of the above. I have few expectations for it being read or thought about, but maybe one or two readers will happen upon it and be positively influenced.

I have been a doctor for 57 years and a Physician for far less. This series of essays describes my consternations and tribulations while becoming a Physician, my concerns on the business aspects of practicing medicine, and my views on the differences between being a Doctor of Medicine and a Physician. They are presented in three sections, with the essays in each focusing on those subjects. They may express the frustrations experienced in my years of practice, but they cannot communicate the joy, pride, and satisfaction I have experienced while being a Physician and working with others in the field.

1 Because I hold the idea and the role of the Physician in such honor, I have chosen to capitalize the term where I consider it to be appropriate throughout this book.

2 In this book, 'doctor of medicine' is used to describe both allopathic (MD) and osteopathic (DO) trained doctors.

Readers may gain insight into the dilemmas facing the Physician in practice. Practicing doctors and potential students may be inspired to observe their work more carefully and make improvements in how they perform their professional roles. Some may see the negative effects of the increasingly controlled aspects of medical care. In addition, some may read and decide medicine is not the field for them. If one person benefits in even one of these ways, I will be pleased.

Acknowledgements

There are many people who have shaped my career in medicine, too many to recount. Many have left this world and those who remain will not likely see this work. They led me down this path through advice, example, deed, or act. I shall be ever grateful. I entered medicine to solve problems that disease presented mankind, and I have tried to contribute to the knowledge of medicine. As I fade from my life's professional stage, I see that I ended my career combating disease one person at a time. It was a wonderful journey. I thank those who mentored me.

There are others who played an important role in completing this project. The advice of Leta Waugh at Scribendi helped mold my thoughts and words. Jennifer Stimson's layout and cover design created a pleasing professional presentation for the work far beyond my expectations.

Most importantly, this book would not have existed without the constant support of my wife, Dana. She has supported my avocation, urged me along the path, and reviewed my work. It would not be presentable without her assistance.

Essays on the Practice of Medicine

SECTION ONE

Learning The Ropes –

INTRODUCTION TO SECTION ONE

For 28 years of my professional work, I was a private practitioner caring for patients with pulmonary, critical care, or sleep problems. For many of these seriously ill patients, I, like most in our specialty, would become their primary care doctor, or at least their doctor of first resort when problems arose. In my practice, and I am sure for those in similar work, multiple issues would be placed in my way daily. The situations not only involved caring for patients but also included office, professional, and hospital issues. It was a stressful environment.

I grew into being a Physician during those years. In the beginning, I was an extremely knowledgeable and somewhat known person in my field, but becoming a Physician takes time and experience. I left a world-famous referral institution and accepted a position in a smaller regional referral center. It was there that I grew into and, I believe, earned the title "Physician."

Now, reflecting on those years, I realize those stresses were just the natural environment for my profession. I wrote these essays in Section One because of that stress. Yes, some doctors have more stress than others, but a Physician responsible for patient care always experiences stress. If a doctor does not experience stress, it is because of unawareness, often resulting from overconfidence, narcissism, ego, intellectual smugness or, dare I say, the lack of a moral compass. These are not good personality traits for a medical doctor to possess.

The essays contained in the first section reflect my observations and feelings during the time I was at the forefront in the war against disease, one patient at a time. Although I no longer practice full time, these issues still affect many of those who do. They include how we, and others, view illnesses and responsibilities, how we judge coworkers and ourselves, and why we continue to work as healers. They represent my experience becoming a Physician. The essays composing Section One were previously published in *Arizona Medicine*. They are used here by permission.

A physician's work and behavior are heavily influenced by his workplace and responsibilities. In Section Two, the essays are on some of those influences that the practicing physician does not control. They reflect a view of medicine as a business that is somewhat dark. Unfortunately, for most doctors, effecting change in the business of medicine is out of reach. Many, but not all, doctors share these often negative views.

In Section Three, I focus on my perception of the differences between a Doctor of Medicine and a Physician. I describe my perception of a Physician. The distinction is my own, but to a patient under a Physician's care the distinction is clearly recognizable. My description is circumstantial and indefinite as the role, wrapped in values, defies specifics. My goal is to provide a clearer vision of what makes a Physician.

The Best Doctor In The World

It seems so obvious to me. Each of us should want to be the best we could possibly be. Is that different for physicians? I think not, but what then is the best we could be? Is there common ground between the neurosurgeon, the radiologist, the cardiologist, and the family physician?

You might think that Doctors of Medicine, with the benefit of their education, experience, economic position, and status, would have an answer to this question. If they were asked, the answer should be quick and clear. I must confess that when the thought first occurred to me, I was many years out of my training and I had not confronted the concept before. Somewhere along that ten-year road of training, it must have belonged. Needless to say, I am not one to shy away from questions, particularly when the answer is not apparent.

"Not apparent"—yes—that is exactly what I meant to say. I did not know the answer to the question, "What is 'The Best Doctor in the World'?" Not only did I not know, I rapidly became aware that to find the answer would take some study. The process has been completed and I wish to share the results of my inquiries.

My colleagues assisted me with their knowledge on the subject. John, a cardiothoracic surgeon, spoke calmly as a man who has experienced much of the world. "To be there opening the chest, to see the heart beating, to stop it, to fix it, to restart it, that is what I do. 'The Best Doctor in the World' should be able to perform heart surgery with speed, skill, grace, and perfection." I pondered his response. Yes, these facts are important. I would want my procedure to be done with speed, skill, grace, and perfection, but somehow I could not accept his definition. It is probably because I am not a surgeon. Obviously, I should have asked an internist.

Sam is an excellent cardiologist. He looked at me suspiciously in response to my question. I could not escape the feeling that he was stalling for time. As he was always quick with the correct diagnosis, it seemed unusual for him to ponder a subject. "'The Best Doctor in the World' is able to assess the situation quickly with a minimum of history, to confirm his suspicions with a brief exam, and to arrive at a plan of action. Accuracy of diagnosis is of the utmost importance. Accuracy of treatment will follow." Yes, that sounded much more to my taste—history, exam, assessment, and then treatment. The age-old, well, eighty-year-old approach—the scientific approach to medicine. Then I remembered my past exposures to the scientific methods of modern medicine. At least my medical school had not let me down.

My joy of discovery must have been evident. Nancy could not suppress her curiosity. "What are you up to?" the nurse inquired. "Researching the attributes of 'The Best Doctor in the World,'" I delightedly confided. Unlike my colleagues, she did not pause to inhale. "That's a piece of cake," she exclaimed. "It is Dr. Wonderful! When we have questions he says, 'Page me.' He writes clearly, he makes rounds early and at the same time every day, and he never complains about phone calls at night for clarification of orders written that morning." A different perspective to be sure. It is something to consider.

My confidence was dipping a bit. Each person I questioned had their own distinctive view of "The Best Doctor in the World." Each view seemed correct in its own right but so different from the others.

"Could the hospital CEO shed some light on my question?" I wondered. Constantly dealing with physicians and medical care issues, he must know the attributes of "The Best Doctor in the World." My appointment with Harold occupied the three o'clock period on Wednesday. He maintained a relaxed air of confidence when meeting with physicians as though it had all happened many times before. He did not seem happy with my question. Unprepared and startled expressions crossed his face. He must have been expecting a request for a zillion dollars' worth of new equipment.

He answered without thinking. "The doctor who admits his patients to St. Us and promptly cures them. But it is not that simple," he continued. "Of course, elective cardiac and orthopedic procedures with effective utilization review and appropriate patient insurance profile provide the maximum revenue return to offset . . ." The words continued, but the meaning, although hidden in business speak, was evident. Different to be sure, but evident.

"Can I be honest with you?" he questioned, drawing my attention from my thoughts. "A hospital CEO loves the 'average' doctor. If all our doctors are too good, then their patients stay healthy and don't need the hospital. If the doctors are too bad, then they admit the patients too soon, keep them too long, and use too many resources. Yes, just give me the 'average' doctor and I'll give you a successful hospital." Now that put the cards on the table for me to see. I wondered, if Harold were to experience an abdominal pain that would curl a Marine into a sobbing child, would it change his view of 'The Best Doctor in the World'?"

Depressed! It was making me depressed. I thought my study would be simple, but each person had his own perception of "The Best Doctor in the World"—none of which seemed to ring true and right with me.

In the middle of my dilemma, Sidney telephoned. "I think I have bronchitis. You know, green sputum, hacking cough, and fever—no chest pain or shortness of breath. Could you call me in an antibiotic? Tomorrow, I need to be at the 'college' meeting to present a paper." Sidney is a doctor. We doctors are like that. Often self-diagnosed and sometimes self-treated. We don't like the "system" and do our best to minimize our personal contact with it.

Smothered in work, I had no time for pondering my obsession. I was falling behind on my schedule, and one long-time patient could not hold his irritation.

"If you guys"—meaning doctors, I interpreted—"were any good, I wouldn't have to come all the way down here and waste my time—not to mention money. We could do this by phone," he blurted out.

"By phone!" I echoed, more startled than irritated.

"Yes, by phone. If you were really good, a few questions and 'blam!' you would know the diagnosis and could call in the treatment," the patient responded—in case I had missed the meaning. I had not.

His point was clear. It would be extremely difficult, if not impossible, to diagnose and treat by history alone. But if you were "The Best Doctor in the World," the best there ever was to be, you could do that. It is what our patients want. It is what we want—just like my friend Sidney. The second-best doctor might require an exam, while a doctor with lesser skills would require invasive tests or treatments or even hospitalization.

My patient knew there were limits to my skills and accepted my failings while wishing for the ultimate in medical care. My patient answered the question I had asked of everyone but him.

A person who seeks assistance with an illness wants a minimum of contact with the system. He wants to be well and stay well. If given the choice, we all would choose to live our lives like Oliver Wendell Holmes' One Hoss Shay in "The Deacon's Masterpiece" and be perfect in every way for 100 years to the day.

"The Best Doctor in the World"—patients and providers each have their views. Ultimately, everyone becomes a patient and we view "The Best Doctor in the World" from that perspective. As a patient, we desire the least medical care necessary to make us well and to keep us well. As a doctor, the same should be true. We should aspire to deliver the least medical care necessary to make our patients well and to keep them well. And to be sure, the medical care we deliver should be our best.

Acts Of God Or Acts Of Man

Questions, questions, questions. . . . Why do I ask myself so many questions? Here on the road, driving home at four a.m., there are other things to think about. But no, I ask myself, "Why? Why? Why?"

The call came as usual just after I was past my point of no return—asleep. You know the point. The one after which you can be awakened, but you really don't awaken until the caffeine level hits red alert.

The situation had sounded all too familiar. The patient was discovered by the nurse with distressed breathing and low blood pressure. She rapidly progressed to full cardiac and respiratory arrest. The emergency team had reacted and performed, as I so often had witnessed, like a premier symphony orchestra and pulled the patient back to the world of the living. Then it was my turn to perform.

It must have been the frustration of it all: one too many nights called out, one too many very sick patients to see, and one too many extraordinary efforts caring for the extremely ill. On other nights my mind did not wander, but that night I asked myself—"Why?"

For several years, our corner of the medical literature had been covered with new insights into causes, mediators, and theories on the patient's problem—sepsis. None of these had changed the basic treatment objectives. While our agents have changed, what we try to achieve with those agents remains the same. No, it was not the "medical" aspects of the problem that troubled me.

My patient fit the mold of the medical problem. She had initially been hospitalized for elective surgery, and the course had been straightforward. The day before the dramatic events in which I participated, there were signs of impending problems. A new fever, an indwelling bladder catheter, and a rising white blood cell count had been observed and noted in the chart. All the appropriate laboratory studies had been ordered, but no one had decided to treat her before the results were returned.

If only someone had . . . ??

As I reflected on the evening's adventure, I was pleased. The sheer beauty of a confident, knowledgeable medical team working together at their life's work was a great thing to have shared. It was like an opera orchestrated and sung for themselves and that one semiconscious patient.

The question would not go away. Why? The day before, if only someone had . . . ? Our private concert, thankfully a success, would not have been needed. Too often the concerts have tragic endings, and they are not the sort of performances for which you or your loved ones would want the central role.

The following morning, Friday, it happened again! I was opening the door to see the 8:30 appointment—it was actually 9:05 and the appointment had been moved up from 10:30—when Helen, my secretary, stopped me. "You are needed on line one. The Intensive Care Unit has blood gases!" she reported. An ICU tradition, it was my third blood gas call that morning.

Now even further behind, I rushed back to my waiting patient, but there was that nagging question again. Why? My plans carefully laid out months in advance were a shambles. Today I was to be teaching at St. Mecca Hospital. Although on my schedule for weeks, it had been overlooked by the staff until yesterday. Then, after discovering the oversight, they spent half a day changing the schedule. The patched-up schedule left everyone unhappy and me late and exhausted.

That evening, as the door to the office closed for the final time, the staff left with their usual, "Have a good weekend!" Quiet at last! Just the afternoon charts to dictate, several messages to answer, and several other charts to read and sign. Almost always, there was work to complete after the staff left. However, tonight the stacks were twice as high as usual. Why, why, why? Obviously an "Act of Man." The failure to notice the change in schedule led to the day's chaos.

It was two days later, late Sunday afternoon, when the question came to me again. My wife and I were shopping at the local mall after my hospital rounds, which occupied the morning and early afternoon. It was a particularly busy day, and I had to answer a pager call every twenty minutes. The questions were usually ones that had already been addressed or should have been addressed on rounds at the hospital that morning and not at the shopping mall. The last ring of the pager released the frustrations of the week. "%#@*& it to *&$#%, what is going on down there today?" I hissed to my wife. After further raving about the intelligence of the pager, I answered the call.

"Doctor, I'm so sorry," she began. "He was fine. I saw him ten minutes before it happened. He was joking and happy, visiting with his family. The code team has been working with him for 20 minutes. They haven't been able to obtain a rhythm or a pressure. I don't know what happened. . . ." She spoke more softly as the urgency left her voice. "I'm so sorry. He was such a nice man."

"I know," was all I could answer.

The same skilled team that revived the unfortunate person of three nights ago was unable to repeat their performance with the "nice man"—a patient and, as most clinicians feel about their longstanding patients, a friend for eight years. Awaiting elective surgery, he had succumbed to a sudden episode of ventricular tachycardia, without identifiable reason or cause.

The question returned. Why, why, why?

It was as if an invisible force had swept down and said, "It's your time." Like an "Act of God" (or gods, or whatever divine entity you envision). It had been decided that it was his time to die, and die he did.

Without warning, his life was over. I reviewed the events of the morning and could identify no fact that should have foretold the impending disaster. Why did it occur and why now? Of course, there are a multitude of medical answers, but it was like an "Act of God"; an event occurring without forewarning, the results appearing inevitable.

The answer to my questioning appears to be a simple one. Events result from "Acts of God" or "Acts of Man." There are events beyond our control and understanding; events that happen for reasons we do not have the knowledge to comprehend. Until we do possess this understanding, these events will remain "Acts of God." More commonly though, we face events that we have the knowledge to understand and the ability to control or alter. These "Acts of Man" may disguise themselves as "Acts of God," but often they are obvious. "Acts of Man" can be as simple as the schedule oversight or as mysterious as the unidentified septic patient, each requiring extraordinary effort and activity to overcome and correct. But each holds in common that a single step by an individual might have prevented the wild events that followed.

Many times as physicians we delude ourselves into thinking our primary role is to combat "Acts of God," but in reality it is the "Acts of Man" that we most often are confronting. A person's self-abuse, a drug or procedure ill-chosen, or a warning sign missed or ignored are all typical "Acts of Man" that a physician must face.

For each event that marks our day, we should consider what we might have done differently that could have prevented or changed the event. Was it an "Act of Man" that we could have altered by a simple stroke of the pen or a different decision? Often it is the small things we overlook in the press of the day that, in retrospect, with attention, may have changed the course of future events.

A bard once said, "Trifles do not make perfection, but perfection is made of trifles." Can we, by attending to the "trifles" of our profession, reduce those "Acts of Man" that plague each of us? I think so.

Links In A Chain

Waves tugged at the moorings. Our boat rocked and jerked as the bow rose with the swells and the mooring chain held it in place. Although protected from the usual westerlies, we lay exposed to the sea on the leeward side of the island.

My mind raced with thoughts of the rocky shore just a few yards away. Sleep did not seem possible despite the exhaustion which follows a long passage. I heard the straining of the lines and the crashing of the waves on the breakers. The lines would growl and squeal as they tightened, but I thought of the chain linking us to the bottom—holding us in place. It was our link to the earth, our handhold to our world, a chain that looked as old as the island itself. How good was it?

Sleep did come, and it was the sleep sailors learn to long for in harbor—quiet, long, and deep. Experience has since taught me that, to a "real" sailor, the event would have been just another day's sail and anchorage, but to me it was more. For I was not a "real" sailor.

On another beautiful morning, after a leisurely breakfast with my wife, I started rounds late. "Where were you?" the nurse demanded. "The answering service said you could not be found! This patient's oxygen level dropped and we needed help. Fortunately, when they couldn't find you, I found your partner making rounds and he took care of the patient!"

Her attack on my professionalism left me defensive and irritated. The facts of the morning turned out to support the nurse's tirade on my professionalism. An early morning call was placed to the office and forwarded to my answering service. Since at the hour of the call I was usually on my pager, the service did not try to reach me at home. When the nurse called a second time, the irritated answering service operator exclaimed, "We can't find him." Because of a leisurely breakfast and the presence of an irritated operator, my professionalism was labelled by one nurse, at least, as substandard. A link in my coverage had broken.

I have experienced other times when the integrity of an inanimate object tied me to the ground. All of us have. The rig was in the western high plains of Oklahoma. We were pulling pipe from an 11,000-foot hole in the field just southeast of Corn. The summer sun had baked the ground and us to a golden brown. As I climbed on the platform, my head still ached from the nitro we had used in cutting the pipe. Charlie had sliced the pipe clean with the nitro blast and he had worked it free with our hydraulic jacks. All that was left was to pull the pipe.

Pulling the pipe in the oil fields was a summer job for me. For Charlie and the others of the crew, it was their full-time occupation. I worked the floor, which at Corn was seven feet off the ground. My role included loosening the joints with a four-foot wrench and several licks from a sledge. The wrench rotated the pipe by being tugged with a one-inch rope over a winch. Halfway through pulling the pipe, with one very stubborn joint, the rope snapped. The wrench, swinging free, caught me under the right shoulder blade and lifted me off the floor into the air. I can still see the horizon and the rig in slow motion as I fell to the ground below. A link had snapped. Only my pride was hurt, but a lifelong lesson was learned.

Another time, my holiday had passed at home with relatives unseen for years. We enjoyed our time in a storybook fashion. Upon checking in that Sunday night, I was informed by my partner that one of my regular patients had become ill and required hospitalization during my absence.

Like many physicians who know their patients well, I was not surprised by the events that had led to the hospitalization. They could not have been less storybook-like. A sudden onset of fever, followed by increasing cough and shortness of breath, led the patient to start her home antibiotic program, but she progressively deteriorated with the onset of chest pain and labored breathing. Frightened, she had called our service and was ultimately hospitalized.

"Have a good time?" she beamed. I have always been amazed at the ability of a positive personality to show through any hardship. This patient's personality was "positivity plus." Her smile crossed from cheek to cheek under her oxygen and between the coughs.

"Why, yes," I replied, somewhat surprised at her countenance. "How are you doing?"

"Wonderful! Well, much better at least, thanks to . . . ," she continued. The first on her list was the helpful lady at our service. Then came my partner and the others whom we might expect on the list. This time the links held firm. There was no gap in the care of my patient.

I'm a little more experienced now in the ways of seamanship and medicine. When anchoring, I automatically inspect the chain and rode as it plays out. Sleep comes easily and refreshes.

My medical chains are not played out as dramatically. No dropping anchor to watch, but the links are there and no less important. As physicians, we have assumed the role of caregiver to those who have entrusted us with their lives—even when the office is closed or our girl "Friday" is off, when we celebrate with our loved ones, and when we do the hundreds of other things we do. Who do our patients call? Where do they go for help? And who cares for them in our absence? These are the links in our care. Links we must inspect to ensure their integrity.

The welfare of our patients depends upon the links in our chain of care. In our profession, these links are as important to our patients' health as the chain and anchor are to the boat's safety from the rocky shore. It is said that a chain is only as good as its weakest link. Our chains are no different. Have you inspected your links of care lately?

Responsibilities

The medical record lay open on the desk as the evening shift records clerk and I looked at it together. The saga of this record was a story itself. Now, it was here for me to dictate the discharge summary. I had summoned the clerk to ask why. The patient's five-week hospitalization had been a story of success and failure, joy and misery, and ultimately relief and release from the disease and hospital. I had played a supporting role in the cast of characters along with other physicians.

The clerk, new in the medical records department, appeared nervous. The record had made the rounds to several of the participating physicians before my visit. Each had passed it on to the next; some, even those primarily responsible for the care, saying that the summary was not their responsibility, while others just ignored the issue. The discharge summary is normally a responsibility of the admitting physician, but in this case the admitting physician had little to do with the patient's care.

"He asked me to ask you if you would mind doing the discharge summary," she offered. The hair on the back of my neck raised. My immediate thought was to tell her to tell . . . well, you know the thoughts. Fortunately, an attack of rationality got its hold on me before my mouth opened. The attending just needed help getting a reasonable summary of the hospital events done. "OK," I answered. I dictated the discharge summary.

Experience has taught me some things are better just done than thought about, talked about, or dodged. The time spent and the frustration experienced can both be greatly reduced by recognizing when accepting responsibility is appropriate. I wasn't always comfortable accepting responsibilities.

I can still see the lamp as it crashed to the floor, shattering into fragments. Although my share of the blame should have been clear and obvious when judged by the historical records of that year, the phrase, "She did it!" came from my lips. My sister and I were playing, actually fighting, in the one room in which we were not to play or fight. The lamp's flight and landing represented a casualty of the main round.

Our mother was extremely tolerant by nature, but the loss of one of her few "nice things" was not taken well. After reviewing the facts, somehow my words, "She did it," did not shift the responsibility in her eyes. Punishment was swift and probably less than deserved.

My initial experience with clinicians and responsibility came on my first rotation as a junior medical student. I was fatigued and weary after a night on call, and it was time for rounds with the attending. This professor, who had a reputation that put Attila the Hun to shame, was rumored to eat students for breakfast. His first question was benign enough: "Any interesting admissions last night?" I thought of my patient, and while I was considering the merits of going one-on-one with Attila, my friend and partner spoke first.

"Why, yes, sir," he said with enthusiasm. The case description came next. The feeling of relief that came over me had to be similar to the relief felt by the condemned hearing the pardon. As my attention refocused on the situation at hand, the case seemed very familiar. It was at this point I realized what my friend was saying. "His presentation was unique, but Bob, it was your case, so why don't you tell Dr. Attila about it?" Talk about slick. I had received my first responsibility "turf." I survived and was wiser for the experience. Now I foresee and handle those "turfs" better.

"He said what?" I questioned the nurse. She had passed the message about an extremely ill patient from another consultant whom I did not know.

"He said to tell you to get this man off the ventilator and extubated," she responded, and after a long pause added, "today."

Obvious and worthy goals for an intubated ventilated patient to be sure, but the patient still required total support from the ventilator and would not survive without it. A call to the physician told me more. His frustration with the lack of progress the patient and his portion of the patient's problems were making became evident. Since he was doing everything he knew to do, it seemed to him that the ventilator was holding up any progress in the recovery of the patient. Therefore, it was my responsibility. Often we shift responsibility when the events do not go as we have planned or promised.

My interactions with other clinicians often lead me to reflect upon our responsibilities. Responsibility is often relative and overlapping, not just absolutely ours or theirs. Those are obvious. The shared ones are where difficulties arise. We each tend to perceive our share differently. The complexities of our applied science contribute to this problem of perception. Most disease ends up affecting the whole and not just the parts. It is hard to draw exact lines separating responsibilities for ourselves and others to see.

In the course of illness, the path is never sure. Nature can redirect it. Our attempts at altering the path can lead to unexpected changes and dangers, while oversights or inattention to care may divert it. Reacting to these changes, we can assess them with open minds, attempting to understand what they are, why they happened, and what our role was in their creation or evolution. When physicians accept these responsibilities, better care is the result. But when we are too eager to assign responsibility to the patient and his lifestyle, to the disease, or to others involved in the patient's care, discord results and patients suffer.

Caring for the same patients, physicians who can assess, understand, and accept responsibilities perform in harmony, with overlapping melodies and blended chords. Or, as is too often the case, when we cannot, do not, or will not, a clamoring of noise and discord erupts. Generally, the harmony of care is experienced and heard by all who care to listen. Patients, physicians, nurses, staff, and others all reflect the music being played. How are your melodies being heard?

Attitude

It was one of my first experiences interviewing for a position as a physician. Although fully trained and "boarded" in my field of interest, I was still relatively young and inexperienced. After asking to see some patients with them, I was rounding with the senior member of the group to learn about their practice and techniques. Coming to the first patient, he leaned to me in a confidential manner and confided, "This old lunger is a drunk."

Having spent time training in county, V.A., and military hospitals, I was more than familiar with the medical and social problems associated with alcohol excesses. No matter—I was startled at his comment.

As the afternoon progressed, I learned that he characterized most of his patients in similar derogatory terms. The more difficult the management problem, the more shrill became the descriptions. Earlier he had seemed courteous, pleasant, and thoughtful, but clearly his approach to patient care was unhappy at best. I didn't take the job.

Daily events often reveal our approach to life. My new VCR started to eat tapes when we played the third tape, yes, the third tape. It was also my third week of ownership. The warranty instructions were explicit. Problems during the first 90 days and off to the service center it goes. With hope in my heart, I called the store.

The salesman remembered me and the sale. I explained my third tape in the third week story and asked what he thought. "It should not have happened. It is just unacceptable. Bring that VCR down here and we will exchange it for another," he said with conviction.

They did just that and I was overjoyed. Now, I am a faithful customer.

A California physician and I were reviewing health reform issues raised at a seminar we were attending. "We can all cut back a little bit," he explained. I did not understand his comment and told him so.

"We all do things, you know, procedures and tests that needn't be done, but just do them because someone will pay us for them," he explained.

A form of nonverbal communication must have told him my feelings about his comments, since before I could decide how to respond, he added emphatically, "Sure we do! It's human nature. I see it all the time."

As I flew home, the conversation haunted me. In my experience, I too had seen over-utilization without obvious reasons except for economics. Fortunately, such events don't occur among my circle of colleagues.

The stranger had communicated well. Not so much what he said about reform, but rather what he said about his "attitude."

It has become popular to say, "He has an attitude," when someone has obvious strong personality traits. But we all have "attitude." It varies day to day, but does it change at all? My California acquaintance, my video store clerk, and my first interviewer communicated their attitudes well.

Our attitudes shine brightly so that all can see and react. I suspect we all share similar attitudes but in different degrees and combinations. As a result, we are all different. Each of us seems to have one or two attitudes that stand out as ours. Since we all share similar attitudes, we recognize and react to the attitudes of others. Like chameleons, we mirror some. Hostility, happiness, enthusiasm, and joy bring out similar responses from those who meet us. While other attitudes result in opposite reactions. Those that blame, deceive, or are dishonest raise our guard, or should.

As physicians, does this matter to us? I think so.

Medicine remains more art than science. The human role for physicians as healers will remain forever. As knowledge and science progress in the understanding of illness and disease, the role of the physician remains the same. Physicians no longer confront the Black Plague, but many other adversaries have taken its place. As knowledge and understanding of disease improve, responsibilities for treatment can be delegated to others. When a disease is fully understood, preventive measures may eliminate it. In the face of this progress, physicians are busier than ever.

At the front lines in the war against disease, physicians fight battles one on one, each enemy as it is seen and discovered. The battleground is within the patient, the patient whose attitude affects his care and reflects the attitude of his physicians. Could it be that patients who are hostile, frightened, or distrusting are reflecting the attitudes they see in their physicians? Could their fears reflect the insecurity they sense? Just as likely, a patient who is confident he will recover—confident in his care and in his physicians—is reflecting the attitudes of his physicians.

What attitudes do your patients have and project? Certainly not all of these are a reflection of you as a physician, but is there a pattern? Are there a lot of happy, sad, or angry people in your practice? Does this reflect your attitude?

What do our patients see in our attitude? Does it help or hurt their care? We should choose and project the attitude that benefits them. I suspect that the attitude that is best for them will be good for us. When we play the role of physician, our performance affects their lives and our own. Let's get an attitude.

Success

He looked grim as we sat around the table in the lounge. "I don't know if I'll ever get all these patients seen, " he reported. "Two hospitals down and three to go." He waited patiently for a response. Having heard this all before, most of us just ignored the comments.

One relatively new physician could not contain himself. "FIVE HOSPITALS?" he blurted out.

"If I'm lucky, I can be done by seven," the first doctor answered, wearing the obligations proudly. The experienced physicians recognized the participants—the "overworked and proud of it doctor" and his "oh, my gosh" audience—and moved to other things.

Often we relish the activity of our work, with the life and death decisions and their consequences. These times were the dreams of our youth and the responsibilities we sought for so long. With time, the relish and enjoyment mellow. Still a thrill, smaller doses fill the need. Having experienced them, we find that talking about them cheapens the memories of our triumphs and failures. No list of numbers is needed, but we do need some measure of our success, some indicator we are doing what we set out to do.

Since our first days as a doctor, we identified things to mark our progress—signs of success. One of the first I recognized was the call to help a patient. "Dr. Wonderful, Dr. Wonderful," the hospital page would call for all to hear. They were important calls for new physicians—a sign of success. Now, when I hear a page or a beeper shouting "BEEP BEEP BEEP BEEP," I know they are important calls for busy physicians, but I can't help thinking of how we measure success. Is it like notches on a gun handle?

Notches? Yes, notches. As a medical beginner, pages signified being needed. Important physicians were needed to do important tasks for ill patients—to the beginner, a notch of success. Now, as a seasoned practitioner, pages signify something very different. Most pages are not for important changes in patients or to reach other doctors. Rather, most pages come when we forget something, overlook something, or when we asked to be paged. Oh, to be sure, important messages are communicated with the page as a link, but more often it is a confirmation of those feelings of being needed, of being a success—notches on the handle.

What are those notches for? What do they signify? Performance, I presume. Don't we have other ways to perform? I think so.

Performance is as much a part of our "practice" as science. Each act we do includes a performance: the demand "SCALPEL!" for the outstretched hand, lecturing the "students," rounding with the nurse, talking with the family, publishing an article, and the list goes on. It includes the traditional, the professional, and the show. Acts traditional and professional lend credence to our roles as a physician. The doctor's "look" and the steps of listening and examining—they reassure our patients we are professionals and schooled in our art. But sometimes it is just show.

Parading our list of patients waiting to see us, publishing that article, and requesting to be paged all may fit into the category of show: performances more for our ego's benefit than for that of our patients. More notches on the handle that reassure us that we are a success.

In the Old West, the notorious gun fighters would notch the handles of their guns to mark another victim. A measure of sorts, it marked their success. Meanwhile, the Marshall would just do what had to be done and tell the folks, "The show's over. Now go on about your business." He had no notches, no bravado, no attention—just respect.

What does a physician use as a measure of success? Do we confuse the notches on the handle with success? How do we measure ourselves? Where did we learn the scale?

Is it having a long list, a busy practice, an excellent income, the sickest patients, the unique procedure, the most procedures, the most admissions, the . . . ? I think not.

What is it then? A legend I read, reported by Thomas Cleary in his introduction to Sun Tzu's *The Art of War*, renewed my thinking about success as a physician and prompted my writing these thoughts. It is worthy of repeating.

> "A lord of ancient China once asked his physician, a member of a family of healers, which of them was the most skilled in the art.
>
> The physician, whose reputation was such that his name became synonymous with medical science in China, replied, 'My eldest brother sees the spirit of sickness and removes it before it takes shape, so his name does not get out of the house.'"
>
> 'My elder brother cures sickness when it is still extremely minute, so his name does not get out of the neighborhood.'

> 'As for me, I puncture veins, prescribe potions, and massage skin, so from time to time my name gets out, and is heard among the lords.'"

The story relates how early recognition and knowledge of a problem results in quiet success—success recognized only by those involved, not by the world. The success our patients would wish for us when caring for them.

I know we each judge our own success by standards we set for ourselves. Do we realize what these standards are? Do we raise our standards as we approach them so they stay just out of our reach? As physicians, I think we should know what success means to us and work toward those goals.

Have you thought about "success?" What is it to you? Are you content "seeing the spirit of sickness and removing it... ?" Or, have your goals become hazy, or worse yet, notches on a handle?

Tools

I lost my hammer at the side of Highway 9, just east of Norman, Oklahoma. It was the impatience of youth. As I was driving to see my girl at her college, my tire went flat. To get to the spare tire, I took my toolbox out of the trunk and just never put it back. I loved that hammer, and losing it taught me a lot.

Now my tools are more sophisticated, more technical, and more expensive. At one end of the scale, there is my "Latham" stethoscope, which I use three or four days a month. Although 24 years old, it is still my best stethoscope. Since it is hefty and awkward, I have to want to carry it, but I never leave it at the nursing stations. I remember my hammer.

At the other end of the scale, there is my computer and there is my hospital. They each fit one definition of a tool—anything used as a means of accomplishing a task or purpose. My hammer drove 16-penny nails with ease. My computer corrects my spelling and lets me write these words. My hospital helps me take care of my patients. These tools are for my work—and past work—and all require my guidance, follow my directions, and need my knowledge to be of value.

When I first reported to my summer job as a carpenter's helper, I took my "hand-me-down" hammer. The foreman, a man of considerable presence, size, and attitude, looked at my hand-me-down hammer and laughed. "Boy, where did you get that toy?" he asked. The lecture that followed, one of many in my career as a "rough-in" carpenter, told me that better equipment was in order. I finished the experience with the earned respect of the "real" carpenters and with my new hammer—a hammer with character, my trophy of a job accomplished. I was asked back the next year.

Early that first summer, the hammer acquired the first sign of use—its first installment of character. The handle was marked, more a scar or gouge, when I stretched to nail a joist in place and missed. The hammer and joist went flying. By the end of summer I had learned how to use it. Instead of taking eight strokes to drive a nail, a quick three put it in place. In truth, I had been a little wild with that hammer at first.

Hammers, stethoscopes, and computers are tools everyone recognizes, but hospitals?

In the current use of our language, the term "hospital" is used only by those involved in patient care. Hospital and insurance executives long ago decided they were in the "healthcare" business. When caring for a sick patient, physicians need to admit them to a hospital, not to a healthcare business. In a hospital, we can order the tests to diagnose a patient's condition and the therapy to make him well, or at least better.

An amazing array of procedures, therapies, assistance, and care can be mobilized. There are specialized care practitioners in more fields than we can count. Hospitals are buildings, marvels of the twentieth century, designed to deliver quickly and efficiently to the bedside everything but warm food. They are made of brick and mortar, but they, unlike my hammer, stethoscope, and computer, are much more than an arrangement of metal, plastic, and rubber—powered by electricity or not. Hospitals are the people who work there, the living tools who serve the patients at the directions of the physician.

Yes, a hospital is a tool—a tool that only a few have the privilege to use.

Tools benefit from care and attention. Hospitals are no different. The care and attention required for a tool of human form differs from that required by a hammer or stethoscope. The care and attention for a human tool must focus on principles, purpose, goals, and growth—guidance for the future.

Like my hammer, hospitals bear the scars of the new and eager who reach too far with too little experience: scars brought on by business schemes designed by administrators and our colleagues alike. Their scars are bigger than those on my hammer and far more expensive. We physicians often feel that hospital executives (those constant plotters) manipulate our future and pursue the building of empires. We have fostered those opinions by watching their failures and by being able to say, "I told you so." But where were our profession's best and brightest when these schemes were conceived and delivered?

While there is no shortage of hospital critics among our ranks, there is a constant shortage of physicians to provide the care and attention that hospitals need in order to grow. Care and attention are needed for the tool to work as it was designed—to care for sick human beings—and to grow and change like all things human. It is not an easy task. Just as the child may not seek the advice of a parent, the advice and counsel of physicians may not be wanted, may not be popular, and may not be happily received.

Have we been too busy with our professional and personal interests to provide the care and attention our hospitals needed for their direction and growth? I think so. Physician influence is needed now more than ever. Hospital growth occurs daily and needs the wisdom and knowledge that experienced physicians can give: physicians who can focus their attention on the appropriate purpose and goals for our patients and communities; physicians who are concerned about how the tool works and not about building empires, being the first, or doing the most; and physicians simply helping it be the best it can be.

Unlike my hammer, our hospitals will not be left by the side of the road. However, they may leave us—their practicing physicians—and much more tragically, they may leave our patients. Our hospitals have become part of the "healthcare" industry.

The Telephone Call

R-i-n-n-n-g . . . !

"The second ring? I'd better get that now. What's going on? Where is it? Time to get up already? Did the alarm shut itself off?" My thoughts echoed through the void.

R-i-n-n-n-g . . . !

"Now that is the second ring." Awakening enough to know the sound of the phone and to know I'm in bed, I reach for the phone. "Yes?" I answer.

"Doctor, answering service," Kay replies. "I have the hospital again. They need to talk to you about Mr. S. I'll connect you."

"Doctor, Mr. S. is having difficulty with . . . ," the nurse begins to explain. I listen, trying to sort out the facts that don't seem to add up.

Am I on call tonight? Is it still Monday night? My thoughts wander while her voice fades into a void.

The voice doesn't go away, so I struggle out of my semi-stupor and interrupt her. "What's going on? Could you start over?" I ask. Again the story is told. Now the facts make sense, but something is still not right. "Who is Mr. S.?" I ask, getting more basic. The clock reads 12:40 a.m. Surely it must be later.

She explains more about the patient, a professional summary of why he was in the hospital and a background of his case. It doesn't sound familiar, and the patient is very ill and unstable. My mind starts to race. Why didn't I know about this patient? How could I have missed this problem when my partners checked out for the night?

Now fully awake, I question the nurse more about the unfamiliar patient, and finally the answer becomes clear to us both. I am the wrong doctor! The patient belongs to another physician. She apologizes for calling me by mistake, and we hang up. It is 12:46 a.m.

Awake, I remember the first call of the night. Also from the service, it had been only half an hour earlier. But it was different. It was a call for me.

With that first call, the facts added up. The questions about the patient made sense. The answers were easy, and I am not sure if I was really completely awake when I dealt with it. My ability to understand the problem and to respond gave me a level of comfort that allowed me to hang up the phone and go back to sleep.

There is a second sense to being a physician, a sense that picks out the irregularities, the facts that don't add up. It focuses one's attention to identify the important issues and puts them into the right places. When calls come at night, sleep must be interrupted in order to deal with them. Usually they can be dealt with easily and calmly, thanks to our knowledge and experience. Sleep returns and the night goes on.

Sometimes things don't add up, but the confusion still must be resolved. That second sense kicks in, and an adrenalin rush occurs. You become alert and do what must be done. Sometimes, resolving the problem is just as simple as tonight—identifying that the patient belongs to someone else. Other times, more is required.

Simple events often cause me to reflect on things, and tonight had that effect. I've decided that being a physician has a lot to do with learning to listen—and learning when to wake up.

But unfortunately, when the telephone rings at night, once really awake, you are awake. I think I'll try to go to sleep again. It's 2:04 a.m., too early to start the day.

Mrs. B And The Art Of Medicine

She found my name in the Yellow Pages, not the most prestigious source of referrals, but often the one resulting in the most interesting patients. Although she was small of stature, her voice and words refuted both her size and obvious age. Her words of greeting, her gait, her posture, her dress, her diction, all were professionally noted as I became acquainted with Mrs. B.

As physicians, our medical evaluation starts with our patients' characteristics and backgrounds. We hope for sharp separations, clear categories, definable groups—the distinctions we are comfortable with and distinctions we can categorize to help with our diagnoses.

Young of voice and clear of mind, she had lived many good years, and, like most patients when we attempt to classify them, she crossed many boundaries. Now, a troublesome cough had brought her to my office. A mycobacterial infection such as tuberculosis became my primary suspicion, and soon acid-fast bacilli were found on smears of her sputum.

Medicine, we have been taught, is a science. Acceptance of medicine as a science has led to an increasingly factual approach to medical care. With enough observations, studies, experiments, and investigations, we believe that the facts of a disease will be defined. Medicine has achieved this absolute knowledge of some diseases, which can now be prevented or easily cured. Unfortunately, they are few in number. Certainly, much is known, but facts and factors change because our points of view shift, new facts are discovered, or the nature of disease changes.

"Well . . . ," she asked, with her voice fading off, ". . . is it TB?"

"I don't know," I responded. "It may be."

Several mycobacteria can produce positive acid-fast bacterial smears. Some of them cause disease and some do not. I began to explain the various types of mycobacterial diseases but could tell she was still ruminating on tuberculosis.

"So you think it is TB?" she interrupted my explanations.

"I think you have tuberculosis, but we won't know for several days," I added.

Few diseases have such clearly defined steps in their diagnoses and treatments as pulmonary tuberculosis. A patient becomes suspected of having the disease from clinical clues. A culture of the sputum confirms the diagnosis, and well-defined treatment is carried out. The steps in the diagnosis and treatment are clear and clean, sharply defined. But are they?

A few days later, mycobacterium tuberculosis grew in Mrs. B.'s sputum culture, confirming a diagnosis of TB.

Therapy for pulmonary TB requires several drugs taken for a specific time and sequence to cure the disease. Fortunately, a cure is highly likely with the proper medications.

I carefully explained to her the importance of multiple drugs and the required length of therapy. Unfortunately, she did not tolerate the medicines well and started having difficulties her first week.

"Are you sure these are going to make me well?" she asked with a penetrating look. "I feel worse now than ever!" Her liver enzymes had climbed but within acceptable limits.

The facts known about tuberculosis define the disease and the infection for the most part. It is the application of the facts that can prove to be a challenge. Caring for an ill person requires more than a knowledge of the facts.

Only three weeks into her six-month course of treatment taking three antituberculosis drugs, Mrs. B. called one night because of a new skin rash. An allergic drug reaction appeared to be certain. After stopping all her medications, we treated the reaction and then began restarting the medications one at a time.

On each visit, while we worked through the problems with the anti-tuberculosis drugs, her penetrating look became more and more questioning. She asked each time, "Are you going to make me well?" And occasionally she added with emphasis, "Are you *sure*?"

Mrs. B. is better now, well into the treatment of her curable disease. Unfortunately, many illnesses are not so curable, so treatable, and so well defined factually. Caring for individuals with those illnesses, helping with their problems, and directing their treatments often become even more difficult, involved, and time consuming.

So much of what physicians do involves communicating with our patients, herding them along the trail that the facts tell us to follow. I've been down this trail before, the one I'm traveling with Mrs. B., and each time at trail's end, we both realize it has been quite a journey and often quite an adventure.

The trail markers become clearer each year, a contribution of medical science. The scientific facts are important, but have they been given too much significance? Along the trail, there are stretches where we are on our own, the physician and the patient. Places where judgement, instinct, experience, and trust are required.

Of course, change is constant. The trails and the trail markers don't remain the same, so it is important to travel them often enough to stay familiar with the path. Constantly, older facts, laws, and methods are being replaced with new ones.

Now the public has joined physicians as believers in the scientific practice of medicine, believers in practicing by the facts, and believers in the factual trail of medical care. It is an innocent assumption that the practice of medicine is a science rather than an art, an application of facts to a diagnosis rather than the leading of an individual through a crisis of living or dying. But the assumption has led to impersonalized care by many physicians and the advent of large businesses trying to do what physicians do.

The practice of medicine is more than a science. Although a systematic approach to medical problems is essential and regimentation valuable, a flexible approach adapted to the individual remains a must for the appropriate care of most patients. Guiding someone along the fact-lined trail of medical science, helping them know where they have been, and giving them an idea of where they are going—these are the essence of being a physician, the art of medicine.

The Picard Syndrome

A change in television programming last year led me to a new discovery. It did not strike me at first, but it came to me slowly. In fact, I'm sure my insight is already well recognized by others, but in case you're not aware of the "Picard Syndrome," I want to bring it to your attention. It affects so many that we should be fully versed in its many manifestations.

The programming change led to my first significant exposure to "Star Trek, The Next Generation," a show concerning the "Voyages of the Federation Star Ship Enterprise," as the stalwart Captain Picard and his crew explore the Universe. Naturally, a regular assortment of aliens, disasters (natural and otherwise), and crises occur. And not surprisingly, these are dispatched with bravery, stoicism, humor, and unbelievable technical skill by the loyal crew.

Loyalty—the crew has it to spare. A burning alien ship about to explode in deepest space should be enough to scare any sensible person off to the next galaxy. Right? Wrong. If the captain says to go and take a look, the crew rushes off to check out the disaster in the making. What loyalty! What trust!

Crisis after crisis, situation after situation, our captain reviews the data, assesses the options, makes a decision, and off goes the crew . . . all in a matter of seconds. The crew does what must be done: accomplishes the impossible and fulfills the captain's trust in their abilities. Impossible tasks are performed using the space-age equivalent of baling wire and string. These are all done on Captain Picard's order, "Make it so!"

Unbelievable! Am I being overly critical? No, I don't mean to be. Science fiction is, of course, just science fiction. All the technical stuff is just imagination. And I think good imagination is just good imagination. We all had it once. I love it. However, Captain Picard reminds me of too many real people who do not share his fictional expertise but who do have important responsibilities and share his behavior.

As the stories unfold, Captain Picard will be presented with several proposals to solve some complex technical, social, psychological, or philosophic space-age problem. He ponders a few seconds, asks a question or two, and makes his judgment. Then, having sent the crew to carry out the order, he sits back and waits for the next crisis.

His way is the way we would all like to operate: master of our ship, leader of our crew, the recognized decision maker, the one to whom the information is given, to whom ideas are presented, to whom respect is given when a decision is reached, and whose authority is never questioned. There is no need to dirty the hands figuring out which facts are real, important, or apply to the situation; that is the crew's job.

Each of us knows we are capable of the role. We can stand shoulder to shoulder with the captain and match him decision for decision if we only had the chance. But much more is required. Years of experience and unmatched expertise in many fields are essential. For most of us, appearing in our own personal work of fiction would be the best way to shine as captain.

Oh, if life were only so sweet. To Picard it is standard stuff. His order, "Make it so," is a show trademark. To those in life working with their crew, their staff, their employees, their colleagues, Captain Picard's role should represent a fantasy. But if you work with, for, or like a Captain Picard, you are probably dealing with the Picard Syndrome.

A rush to judge, to always know the answer, to make the decision, to have the need to decide and move on, to have unbelievable expectations, to be impatient for action and results, and to be the person in charge: These are the characteristics of the Picard Syndrome.

Leaders and captains are always needed to make difficult decisions, to make sure difficult decisions are made, to set the direction and tone, and to be responsible. How the role is performed, the qualifications of the leader, and the leader's ability to know his own limitations will separate the real Captain Picards from those with the Picard syndrome—the true leaders from the one who is just in charge.

Unfortunately, too many suffer from the Picard syndrome, playing captain, causing pain to those they lead in families, offices, hospitals, businesses, and global corporations. Is there one or perhaps more with the Picard syndrome in your professional or personal life? Maybe it is time to change the channel.

Quiet Please

"What the hell is wrong with this guy?" My thoughts run over one another as I try to make sense of his case. His problems began simply enough, but it is clear that a crisis is approaching. His respiratory rate is in the forties; he labors to breathe; and while breathing 100% oxygen, his oxygen level is dangerously low.

"You bought a used guitar?" A question booms through the ICU, interrupting my thoughts.

"It's a beauty, but there weren't any strings," answers someone. Thank goodness it is in a softer, more conversational voice.

I refocus my thoughts. The patient, admitted two days earlier, has progressively deteriorated. Have I overlooked something? What are all the possible diagnoses? Is there something different I can do to identify the cause?

"Just bring it with you to work tomorrow and I'll check it out," the first voice blasts out behind me. The conversation has moved to the counter where I'm reviewing the chart. My attention turns to the hubbub of the nursing unit.

"Sally, you working tomorrow?" an inquiring voice interrupts the interruption.

"No, I'll work on . . ." Sally begins, and the conversation swirls around and around as they move about the unit.

As I watch the professional care being given among the hubbub of casual conversation and chit chat, I'm proud to be working with this staff, but a thought keeps coming to my mind: "Quiet please!" My patient's nurse works with attention to me and the patient as I review details and make my plans. It takes extra effort today. Every voice seems to interrupt my thoughts, distract my thinking.

Finally, my time with the patient completed, I turn toward the waiting area to review the coming crisis with the family. In the quiet of the waiting area, we discuss his medical problems, and I prepare them for the events I see looming ahead. Their questions answered for now, I return to the unit. The din of the intensive care area contrasts dramatically with the quiet of the waiting room.

The hubbub continues, ebbing and flowing, leaping and crawling, whispering and shouting through the unit. As I watch the activity swirl around the unit, my pride swells. These people, working in the care of others under stressful, trying conditions, are carrying out their tasks with a casual elegance, with grace, and with a professionalism that should be the envy of any group.

There are those who are too loud and too casual, but that is the case in almost all human endeavors. As children, most learn to respect certain situations, to remain quiet and behave appropriately for the time and place. Fewer now are exposed to churches, schools, and family situations where a degree of decorum is expected. A few of those individuals will be found in almost any situation but are particularly noticed in places where quieter surroundings are appropriate.

Actually, some of it—the noise, hubbub, and conversation in the hospital units—is our fault. Many of these workers model their behavior after the physicians who work these same units. We may be setting the behavioral standards. And physicians make their work seem effortless and easy, often enjoying the comradeship of their fellow workers as they care for their patients. Actually, we make our work look too easy.

Most of our decisions are made with reasoned care, with carefully weighted facts, and with many similar prior experiences gathered over the years against which to judge our ideas and responses. We take the complicated and make it simple, conflicting facts and bring them to a common meaning; we tie together a story, physical observations, and physiological measurements into a single whole. Yes, we do make our work look too easy.

The media has done nothing to make the perceptions of our responsibilities realistic, nor given a measured perception of the effort and skills required to perform our work. Sometimes, neither do we. Pride, bravado, or a desire to be sociable may drive some physicians to act out a television drama.

They pull it off much of the time. Most often, though, to do our work we have to think, concentrate, and analyze before a decision can be reached. I certainly do. Unfortunately, those few physicians who are more concerned about socializing and their image rather than the problems of their patients, may cause both their work and their patients to suffer.

I think hospital and office staffs often imitate our behavior of working, or trying to work, efficiently and effectively while carrying on casual conversations, even frivolous ones. Maybe we should be honored, but if the hubbub I have often observed on hospital units reflects physicians' behavior, then maybe physicians need to look at themselves more closely.

We all adopt our professional behavior at some point. Who knows when? It doesn't just appear one day, for it takes time and experience to develop.

How should we act? Are there guidelines somewhere? Have you thought about it? Maybe we should consider how we work and how we appear when we work. Maybe we need less bravado, fewer grim faces, and a little less of "I'm so right and smart."

How should we act as physicians? That is for each of us to decide. But as for me, I'm trying to be professional, of course. I try to be happy, enthusiastic, and enjoy my work, but being serious when appropriate. I try to give it that extra touch of effort, playing my role as my youthful ideal imagined it should be played.

How about you?

The Ride

When the Hyde-Powell cable car crested the hill at Lombard Street, memories took me back decades to my first ride. This night, the view was striking. The Bay Bridge, outlined with lights, silhouetted the skyline of the financial district: a city alive even in the late hours of the night.

After our evening activities, my friends didn't wait for the cable car. Our work in San Francisco completed, we had dined and visited the Wharf. I turned down the taxi they took back to the hotel, choosing to wait for the cable car. It was worth the wait.

Most sophisticated travelers let the "tourists" experience the cable cars, preferring a taxi or limo for their transportation. Most are in a hurry to get to the next site, the next meal, the next store, or just to bed. I know their feelings, but I'm obsessed with a ride I took all those years ago.

I am glad I waited that late autumn evening. The line stretched out, but the wait was not long. As usual, a local balladeer serenaded those of us in line.

After my friends left, mostly couples remained, and they crowded the seating as we boarded. Despite the line, the car would not be full. As I approached, my place remained open.

I always try to get the same place, my place, when I ride—an outside standing position at the very front of the car—the place to catch the air first and see the views ahead. You can rest one leg on the front rail of the car and lean forward to look across to the other side—the best viewpoint in the car.

I had found my place many years before on that prior visit in my early teens. No, my name is not on it, but it is still my place on the car. Of course, others are often in my place when I am there to ride, but not that night.

The joy of having my spot, mixed with the cool breeze and the sound of the car's bell, Clang de la clang . . . clang, clang, clang, was magical. It wasn't until we stopped at the crest of the hill and I saw the Bridge and the City that my senses cleared enough to realize how reassuring it was to ride those cars again.

I am not sure why, but when I was a kid riding the cable cars, I knew I would be back again and again to claim my spot at the front. I would do what had to be done; I would travel there or live there, but I would be back.

I am older now, less sure of the future. Friends have come and gone, died and passed from the scene. My family has changed, and I am twice the age of my parents when I took that first cable car ride. Life appears more uncertain.

I needed a ride that fall night. The cable car provided it and more: a simple cable car line to a single destination. I had a goal, and it took me there as it did so many years ago. But the ride represented more. It represented consistency, reliability, durability: much of what we lack in our current daily experiences.

The wind, the view, and the chill all served to take me back to earlier times . . . to feel alive, to experience the City once again. It served to tie me to a time when things were different, when things were simpler for everyone, when most things were a new joy.

The demagogues say times are different now and we must change. Certainly, with the passing of time, technology produces changes in our world, changes which often confuse our senses and our directions. But mankind, although growing and maturing in many ways, has not changed.

It is still only as individuals that we determine our values, our purposes, our goals: dependable, durable guideposts for us as we travel down to the end of the line. Our individual lives are traveling to a single destination: a trip made easier by knowing the fare, the stops, and the views along the way.

Though I am now far away from the City, I know my place at the front of the car is waiting for my next late night ride. If you travel there before me, take my place in the night air. I hope it carries you back to where you want to go.

Essays on The American Medical System

SECTION TWO

Medicine as a Business –

INTRODUCTION TO SECTION TWO

Being a doctor, a Physician, is an honor. The work is rewarding and stimulating. Becoming a doctor is but the first step in the professional journey of a lifetime; it involves additional training and ultimately a practice or institutional position. And, for better or worse, the work done will be strongly influenced, controlled, and restricted by the business of medicine.

A doctor should work for and with his patients to their benefit. This has been so since the profession began. The essays in Section One reflect some of my trials and tribulations while trying to live up to that standard. Those in Section Three describe the standards of being a Physician. The essays in this section emphasize my concerns with the business of medicine.

A current popular concept is that the doctor's role is for the greater good, society's good, rather than that of the individual patient. This change in concept appears to be spreading throughout large practices, medical schools, and medical specialty societies. It is a political, economic, and business movement.

Doctors are taught to look to the experts for guidance. Medical societies have published "best practice guidelines" for thousands of conditions. Insurance companies have their own payment guidelines that affect how a doctor may practice. These become "best practice guidelines" for doctors in their system. Our government's regulations and commercial insurance corporations' restrictions become guidelines by default. Now, many young doctors are more concerned with fitting patients into a diagnostic box that gives them the guidelines for care than actually assessing what the patient needs: It is work a 1990s computer could do. Doctors are to be foot soldiers in society's war on disease and other ills, society's servants. Individual patients are to be managed solely by the guidelines for their specific medical box. No independent thoughts or reviews are needed. Just apply the guidelines.

The consecrated electronic medical records required by the government enshrine and enforce these goals. They are programed to allow the doctor to choose only A or B options. Other possible options, C through Z, are not even considerations. The electronic record is a major deterrent to allowing the choice of alternative options.

Large corporations, insurance companies, individuals with no healthcare experience, and many types of businesses now often employ doctors. They are employed in all manner of roles in addition to patient care. These employers often have no code of ethics other than their own. The doctors are accountable to administrators, committees, boards, and other groups of individuals also employed by the organization.

As a Physician, I find the changes disheartening. As an older person, I find the changes alarming for the health of my family and myself.

The essays in this section reflect upon the business of medicine in America. Compared to the essays in Section One, their tone is less personal, less optimistic, and more universal. These are my views of the business of medicine from my years in practice: if you will, the infantryman's view of the army. Most infantrymen have opinions on the army's problems and how it should be run. I, as a practicing Physician, am no different.

These essays may tend to cast a negative view on the business of medicine. Some may exaggerate to make a point, but there is truth in each one. Medical care costs too much, and the patients are often totally unaware of the value of what they are receiving. Likewise, physicians often have little concept of the cost of the care they are recommending and providing. Too much money is made by businesses who own health-related activities, businesses that are not responsible for the care of the patient and whose sole aim is profit. Change is slow, but change is coming and is needed. Let's help guide the changes in the best direction.

How Are You Paid?

While in high school and college, I enjoyed my part-time work the most when I was the only one responsible for getting it done. I was paid for doing it, and when I did it well, I was usually paid well. Those times taught me how I expect the system to work. They taught expectations of how I should be paid, which have stayed with me to this day. Now I have to wonder if my expectations fit the future of our profession.

These thoughts came to me after a utilization review nurse called me regarding a hospital patient. "Did you know Mr. Emphysema was on the 'Capitation Plan' in which you don't participate?" she asked. Of course, I didn't know, and I hadn't looked. I had been asked to see the patient, and I did. For three days, I cared for the patient, and he was almost ready for discharge. Yes, it was my responsibility to note the patient's insurance coverage before doing my work, but habits are hard to break.

Early in my practice years, I asked a consultant to see an unstable patient. Late that day, I checked with the nursing unit to assess the patient's situation, only to discover that the consultant had not seen him. I learned he was waiting to clarify the patient's insurance coverage. The patient was doing poorly.

Vowing to never put the insurance coverage and method of payment before the patient, I called another consultant. I never called that first physician to see another patient. My patients have benefitted from this experience, but it has caused me to have this habit of working first and checking business details later: an approach that does not lend itself well to the medicine of current times.

My first experiences with how a physician can be paid occurred when I was a medical house officer. Medicine differed from my earlier experiences. We were paid two ways. Our income, fixed by the level of our training, became a secondary consideration as we learned our new profession. Then, house officers experienced a wide range of work: chaos for a month on one service, followed by humdrum on another. The periods of chaos set the standard for most of our experiences. The work was hard, and we often had no clear endpoint for success. Our work was loosely supervised, but it received much negative attention when "problems" developed. Complications, failures to improve, and deaths were events that prompted that attention. We became aware of a second payment system, a negative system, and established our goals accordingly.

As chaos erupted around us, we fixed our eyes on the end of the rotation. Goal number one became to survive the rotation, preferably without any problems. Probably because of the impatience of youth, the end became defined in terms of hours, shifts, or days.

Our second goal was to discharge or transfer the patient as soon as possible. Missed diagnoses, failures to improve, and complications then became the responsibility of another physician or house officer.

Third, a patient's death was to be avoided if at all possible. During those times, physicians were to do everything possible to prevent death—acknowledging it as part of life and our work was yet to become accepted. Fortunately, attitudes are more realistic now.

The phrases, "Not on my service" and "Not on my shift"—watchwords of the house officers of my time—represented our adaptation to that negative system of payment. We were rewarded for completing our shift with minimal problems. Our focus narrowed to achieve those rewards. Unlike the work of my earlier years, the rewards of medicine as a house officer were different. The focus became to do no wrong rather than to do what was right; to serve the attending, the institution, and science, rather than our patients.

Only after entering practice did I begin to receive the rewards for a job well done that my experiences as a youth had led me to expect. In practice, patients become more than a disease, and their health is as much your concern as theirs. If they are well, you sleep well. If they are not, you spend nights on the phone and in the hospital. We both live better when the patient stays well.

The rewards for practicing medicine differ from those of the physician in training and the work of some institutionally based physicians. While practicing medicine, we can be paid twice for our work—if we allow it. In addition to financial rewards paid for the service we provide, we receive the appreciation of our patients—if we work for them and their benefit.

Many of our colleagues share this perspective, but not all. Some did not grow after their days as a house officer. Some are still mostly concerned about their shift. Some hide in their specialty. Some seek employment to shield them from the responsibilities. Some are concerned about the disease and not the patient. Although not spoken, the watchwords "not on my shift" and "not on my service" remain ingrained in their attitudes.

Governments have controlled and influenced medical practice for thousands of years. Ours is no different. It created the legal structure for physicians to practice medicine and, more recently, for businesses to practice medicine. Now, doctors frequently are salaried, have fixed hours, and work for a business instead of for patients. Executives direct the physicians and determine their rewards—how they are paid. These changes may be a dream come true for physicians and patients, but I cannot help worrying about how physicians are paid. It appears that my days as a house officer are coming around again. I already hear the "not on my . . ." watchwords being spoken.

Businesses are becoming responsible for the care of patients. They speak in terms of "covered lives" and "shared risk." They are taking the "payors" world by storm. Well, I don't want a business to be my doctor, and I like being paid by the people for whom I do the work.

But those changes in Medicare codes are on my desk for review, the landlord called today and plans to start remodeling tomorrow, the staff is due for their annual performance reviews, and Dr. Faithful called to tell me he is quitting practice for a salaried job. There is an important hospital committee at four this afternoon, and for now, I have to go see this urgent consult. I wonder, when will working for the patient not be worth the hassle? Too soon, I fear.

The Make a Car Program

Once upon a time in a galaxy far, far away, free men met to decide their future . . . .

"Individual transportation is a right. We must provide cars," bellowed the assemblyman. On this statement, the "Make a Car" program was born.

Everyone was to drive a car, so a car would be given to each and every citizen over the age of 21. What a great country!

Then clouds started to appear.

Carmakers were building better cars, and more standard features were available. All standards for quality and safety were being met. The cars cost more.

No expense was spared. As for service, well, the cars were more complicated, but new techniques were developed to care for them, at a cost.

As the cars got older, more repairs were needed because each citizen received only one car and they wanted to keep their car running. Often, just before the car had to be taken to the landfill, repairmen would work for hours trying to repair and save that one car"

One day, the very government Assembly that began the "Make a Car" program was working on a "Make a Job" program. To their amazement, they found they were running out of money.

"Horror of horrors, where is all this money being spent? Where is it going? How could we spend so much?" asked the assemblymen. What were they to do? The "Make a Car" program was so successful, but clearly taxes could not be raised. Cuts were needed. Surely there was graft and corruption among the carmakers. They would weed it out. And of course, the government must be overpaying for everything. They would have a look.

Costs continued to climb. "The carmakers just don't know how to make a car economically and efficiently," said the assemblymen. "We will pay them less, and they will learn how to do it."

At first, the citizens took little notice. Only a small fraction of citizens became 21 in any one year, and they were the ones who received new cars without upgraded features. They complained loudly, but they were a small voice. The majority felt sorry for citizens who did not get frills, but with the economy the way it was, they understood some were going to have to make sacrifices.

Unfortunately, the cost of the "Make a Car" program was continuing to climb. "Those repairmen are getting paid too much to maintain the old cars," concluded the assemblymen. "They are making extra repairs and charging us more. We will fix that."

Now, 50 years have passed. In that vast land, all the citizens over 21 have a car, but their cars rarely run.

Yet they must still pay the taxes to pay for the cars because everyone over 21 gets a car from the "Make a Car" program. The cars are cheap and break down soon. The wait for repairs is long.

The citizens want cars, but not from the "Make a Car" program. Unfortunately, they cannot buy different ones because the other carmakers could not compete and went out of business. The citizens are unhappy.

The Assembly is happy. Costs are under control, and the program is working. Everyone gets a car.

They will now be able to add new programs. They have much work to do.

When the assemblymen travel, they have special arrangements for transportation and do not use cars from the "Make a Car" program. The cars from the program break down too often. How could the assemblymen be troubled to wait to have the cars repaired? Their work is too important.

Was anything learned from the experience? Probably not, for now in the assembly it is heard, "Individual health is a right. We must provide medical care." A program for the health of the citizen is one thing. Providing medical care is something else

Every citizen is going to need medical care at some point in time, for illness is an inseparable part of the human experience. The medical care that will be available, when those citizens need it, is being discussed by the Assembly in that galaxy far, far away . . . .

"A Right To Healthcare" – It Is Not That Simple

Yes, I will try to answer your question. I understand your education has led you to believe that healthcare is a right. Why, you ask, did I pause before saying, "It's not that simple"? But if it were, the answer would have to be "No."

First, consider what is meant by the term "healthcare." Like most words, it is likely interpreted differently by almost everyone. The views will run from having clean water and a family doctor available for medical problems, to those that would include anything to do with a person's health. These are widely divergent categories of products and services based on different delivery systems and business models. It is almost impossible to discuss a "right to healthcare" without understanding everything that is included in the discussion—the components of healthcare.

"Healthcare" is not the only term that needs to be defined. What do the promoters mean by the word "right"? Maybe it is best to consider its meaning first.

When right is used as a noun, as it is in a "right to healthcare," common definitions according to Merriam-Webster include these: qualities of moral correctness or moral propriety; something to which someone has a just claim; something that someone may claim as their due; and a cause of truth or justness. The proponents of a "right to healthcare" generally are using the meanings "something to which someone has a just claim or something that someone may claim as their due."

Healthcare has only one definition listed. Merriam-Webster defines it as "efforts to maintain or restore physical, mental, or emotional well-being, especially by trained or licensed professionals." Practically speaking, this definition would essentially cover all aspects of personal and public health. It would include the fields of preventive medicine, public health, and personal medical care along with institutional medical care. Each of these fields is unique in how it is currently organized and delivered, while sharing some common features. The shared features include the need for physical plants of operation, equipment to provide the services, support staff to carry out the services, and a professional staff. These factors are needed in varying quantities and of different types for each of these fields of endeavor.

For clearer understanding, we need to look more specifically at the services included in healthcare. These would include public health services, preventive medicine services (public or individual), individuals' urgent and chronic medical care, and institutional care (hospitalization and similar). We need to consider all the services that might be determined to be healthcare.

Public health is widely practiced throughout most local communities in our country. Public health services maintain and ensure clean water and adequate sewers, track communicable diseases, and advise the population about those diseases. Their services, physical plant, equipment, staff, and professionals are paid for and employed by government units. They are paid for by taxes and by fees for water and sewer services. For the majority of urban areas in this country, these health services are, for all practical purposes, already a right provided by the government. Certainly, there are exceptions for rural and smaller communities, but most citizens already enjoy public health as a government service paid for by their taxes or available for a fee.

Preventive medical services are currently provided by both government operations and individual medical providers. Examples of government services include monitoring new and current medications for problems, providing recommendations for vaccinations, and monitoring of medical devices. Again, the facilities, staff, equipment, and professionals are supplied and paid for by government taxes and fees.

At a more personal level, physicians, other providers, healthcare businesses and employers, medical practices, clinics, hospitals, insurance companies, and businesses may provide guidance and assistance on preventive medical measures that individuals need. These businesses provide the physical plant, staff, equipment, and professional organization needed. The expense for these services is recouped through fees, insurance payments, employers, and other methods. The healthcare provided at this level is the first at which an individual may be responsible for all or part of the cost of the services.

The next component leads further into an individual's responsibility. It is providing their own urgent and ongoing medical care. This is the form of healthcare we are familiar with and what is most often thought of when discussing "a right to healthcare." In our country's history, these services have been provided by individual professionals who own and operate their own businesses. Recent changes in economics, economic policies, and legal structures of medical businesses have led to more large organizations, such as hospitals and insurance companies, owning more of these types of businesses. These operations in any form—the expenses from cotton swabs to physician income—are paid for by individuals, either directly or through surrogates (employers, insurance, or others).

An individual's surrogates are the primary payors for the institutional care portion of the healthcare delivery system. This portion of healthcare, hospitalization primarily, is where the largest cost (facilities, equipment, staff, and professionals) occurs. Again, most of the cost is paid for by individuals or their surrogates.

In the areas of healthcare where the individual is mostly responsible for the cost of the service, there is one major group of individuals that is not directly responsible. Those are individuals on government insurance such as Medicare. In Medicare and other government plans, a person may have a markedly reduced exposure or no exposure at all to the direct cost of the services. Those who argue for a "right to healthcare" would like all services for all citizens to be paid for by the government taxing citizens.

I am reminded of a quote from Thomas Sowell: "Since this is an era when many people are concerned about 'fairness' and 'social justice,' what is your 'fair share' of what some else has worked for?"

A "right to healthcare" should mean everyone has access to and freedom to decide how to obtain their healthcare. At present, I would argue that it is already the case, but it is disappearing rapidly. In reality, the discussion is not the freedom to get healthcare, but getting healthcare for free.

A Line in the Sand

The form has been on my desk for several weeks. I have not decided what to do with it—fill it out and sign it, or toss it in the trash.

I received this credentialing form from a business in Denver. The accompanying letter stated that an insurance company I have worked with for several years had contracted with them to credential physicians. As I read it over, I recognized all the usual questions about training, licensure, malpractice, criminal activities, and drug usage, but near the end there were some new ones. Do I take any prescription drugs? Do I have any continuing health problems? Have I been hospitalized in the last ten years? Who else do I contract with to provide my services for their patients? The answers were easy enough—no, no, no, and . . . but why should they know more about me than I am allowed to know about my employees? While it is easy for me to complete now, will it be so easy five or ten years from now? How do other physicians who have to answer yes, yes, yes feel about giving out this private information?

It represents the problems physicians face daily. When do we say "enough"?

This form struck me as a step too far—a step over the line. I spoke with them by phone. I was informed that the form must be completed, although their deadline has been extended. I am pondering what to do—pondering this change in the rules.

As kids, we played games with rules that were to be followed in order to play fair. Games taught us much of what we expect in life. The rules of our games would occasionally be changed to make the play more exciting, fairer, or, commonly, more to someone's advantage.

In those games, the rules were changed several ways. Sometimes most of the players thought it would be a good idea, sometimes the loudest and strongest kid demanded it, sometimes someone had a copy of the official rules, and sometimes one of the kids owned an essential piece of equipment (i.e., the ball) and demanded the change.

When we didn't agree with the rule change, the line was drawn. We would draw it in the sand and challenge the other kid to step over it. If he did, as often as not, another line would be drawn—back from the first one—and another challenge issued. At some point the new rule was accepted or rejected. It was withdrawn by its backers, or we argued it out. We went along with the new rule, or we went to play with someone else.

Our profession also has to be played by the rules—thousands of rules from hundreds of sources. Change occurs all the time.

Changes in our professional practices come about for many reasons. We change because the views and beliefs of our profession and colleagues change. In patient care, these changes are often based on "scientific information" of some reliability—a rational basis for change.

Not all change in our patient care is rational. In every profession, there are examples of a particularly vocal and influential representative whose views dictate some aspects of that profession's practice, even when rational evidence may contradict his approach. The loudest and strongest often get their way.

In our business affairs as physicians, change has been coming rapidly and often unexpectedly. Changing the rules is allowed if you write the rules or if you own the game. Insurance companies and government agencies write most of the rules and own many of the games. Rational reasons do not seem to be required.

The credentialing form on my desk represents a change in the rules. If I want to play, I have to go along. I drew my line in the sand. I told them where it was and what it meant. They jumped over it. Do I draw another? Do I lower my standards?

When do we say "enough"? Our professional roles as patient advocates and directors of patient care are under constant pressure.

Hospitals change nursing care levels to meet budgetary needs. In each hospital the response to physician concerns sounds similar—"Our institution is adjusting staffing needs to meet current managed care and reimbursement requirements." What happened to patient care needs? Where do I draw that line in the sand?

Insurance companies and hospitals employ case managers to help with patient care. "Doctor, this patient has used up all his DRG time. He needs to go to the skilled nursing facility today," reads the note on the chart attached to the completed paperwork for transfer. What is the purpose of hospitals and skilled nursing units—the care of patients or maximizing revenue? Do case managers have special skills that physicians lack to determine when the patient is ready for less care?

Mail-in pharmacies write me letters about the cost savings of their generic medications (I sense increased pharmacy profit). Hospitals want to control drug use, but they encourage new procedures that result in additional admissions.

Where is my line to be drawn? When does change go too far? How do we decide?

What do we do? Do we play their game or not? Do we give in and play with the new rules? If we don't lower our standards, will there be other games to play?

Will we have to change our sport out of need or disgust? Which one, if any, will be the straw that breaks the camel's back—the one that leads us away from patient care, from medicine, to other pursuits?

Many physicians I know sense these pressures. Others do not.

Could it be that some physicians have become too concerned about making a living and not concerned enough about how we earn it, about whose standards we work under and about who sets the rules of play?

Who is John Galt, anyway?

And regarding my credentialing form, I am not going to play their game. They have crossed my line in the sand.

Boards

The application has been in my briefcase for several weeks, and each time I look at it I get the same feeling. It's not that I am afraid of failing, or maybe it is. A lot of work will be required to pass the board examination for Sleep Medicine. Dedicating the time needed for preparation will require giving up much of my life.

Board certification is a measure of excellence, at least that's what we have all been taught. But does board certification identify the good physician?

Passing the boards has become an expected ritual in our professional careers. When I took my first boards, my mentors told me that, in the future, passing them would be a measure of my abilities. Unfortunately, what was once a sign of excellence has become the minimal entry requirement to practice medicine. Now, hospitals and insurance companies are beginning to control which doctors a patient can visit. Driven by laws and finances, they need a paper certificate to guarantee a doctor's quality.

The application on my desk represents one of the new board examinations. As each new area of biomedical knowledge develops, physicians working within it begin to organize their interests into a specialty association, which eventually develops its own board examination. After meeting the standards set by already established boards and organized medical societies, the new group ultimately joins them and begins dictating policy for its special area of practice, and a cartel is formed.

As the years pass, the field gradually closes. For a while, practicing physicians are allowed to take the board examination. Ultimately though, to become eligible to take the examination, a multi-year training program must be completed, even though someone may have practiced the skills for years.

At times, the standards have been unfair. And what do you think happens when a large number of doctors are excluded, "locked out," from taking board exams in what they view as their area of practice? In the past, the situation occurred when specialty organizations set entrance criteria that automatically prohibited certain training or experience. Why, of course, the excluded doctors banded together and created their own specialty organization with their own board.

Should I fill out the application and spend much of my spare time over the next year preparing? I have to ask myself, "When does taking a board examination mean you are just foolish?"

In my medical career, I have been eligible at some point in time for no less than six separate boards. I am more embarrassed by the fact than proud of it. For three of them, I have taken and passed the exams and for one of those three, a recertification examination. The fourth one I declined to take, and my eligibility expired. I am still eligible to take the exams for the fifth and sixth (new boards that are in the process of tightening up their requirements). Actually, someone is eligible to take a board exam only when his application passes the review and meets the requirements set up by the "board."

My mentors' comments from years gone by are amusing to me now, for I know that passing the boards does not identify a degree of quality, just a level of factual learning. Yes, most physicians of quality have passed board certification, but many quality physicians have not.

Furthermore, some board-certified physicians do not practice quality medicine.

Now, our specialty organizations are instituting board recertification testing to ensure the continuing quality of their specialists. A process, they report, that would only take a year or two to complete every ten years.

I don't envy those who follow in our footsteps.

Who knows what the next fad in board certification will be. Fad? Well, it is not as extreme as it sounds. We have boards for age groups, organ systems, categories of diseases, physical locations, procedures, physician management, symptoms, and sleep. Many—no, most—overlap one another. Sometimes I think that when I grow up I would like to be an adult, pulmonary, airway disease, dyspnea, ICU, bronchoscopic, sleep physician manager specialist.

There seems to be a cycle of endless business generated by the board organizations, their staffs, and the testing business as well as the obligatory board review courses and preparatory material. Are there some self-serving ends in their drive to certify, recertify, and own the license for their special area of medical practice—to be a cartel? How many of the doctors responsible for these boards actually practice medicine rather than teach or work in administration?

Paper examinations have never separated good physicians from bad ones: the reliable from the irresponsible, the meticulous from the sloppy, the persistent from the quitter, the patient from the intolerant, or the honest from the greedy. Examinations only identify those who know current biomedical facts (as believed by the medical aristocracy) and those who can identify the correct answers, not the integrity we all seek in our own physicians.

Yes, yes, I know that facts are important and I'm speaking blasphemy, but facts can change. If there had been board examinations in 1850, would Semmelweis have passed them? I doubt it, because his belief in the value of hand-washing soon was to cost him his professional life. I wonder if Dr. Barry Marshall had a problem passing his boards in the 1980s believing in the silly notion that a bacterium causes ulcers.

Passing the "boards" does not identify a physician of quality because academic competence is just one of the skills physicians must have and certainly not the most important one.

I can't help but think of the Tin Man, Scarecrow, and Lion. Certified by the Wizard of Oz, they each became what they wanted to be. Do boards work like that? I don't think so. While boards are here to stay, and probably rightly so, a certificate of quality they are not.

Physicians are made, but good physicians are made of much more than facts and figures.

"Open the Pod Bay Doors, Hal"[2] Or, A Tool Doctors Should Control

Once I lost a hammer. It was a tool I earned in my youth while working to finance my education. It taught me to respect the tools I use in my work. On a past occasion (30 years ago), I wrote how doctors should view their tools, a major one being hospitals. My hope was that practicing doctors would work to influence those institutions for the better. Oh, such were the dreams of my youth.

Hospitals are now conglomerates operated by boards and individuals steeped in the profit motives common to all corporations. These are boards and individuals who are far removed from our Oath. They are focusing on the growth and profit for the corporate owners, not on the hospital's services or benefits for the community, patients, employees, and doctors that it serves. The hospital is a tool that I believe is lost for the lifetime of most current doctors. Now, a newer tool already widely used is my current concern: the electronic medical record.

This story begins with my Apple IIe. No, it actually begins much earlier than that. It begins my senior year in high school. An opening in my class schedule allowed me to choose a class of my choice. I chose typing. As a result, I had the advantage of being able to type in college, medical school, and even now. My time in high school was

2 From "2001, A Space Odyssey," a movie by Stanley Kubrick released in 1968 to mixed reviews. Now considered one of the greatest and most influential films ever made. These quotes are taken from a section of the movie on a space voyage from Earth to Jupiter where Hal, the human-like computer controlling the flight and the space craft, has locked the human astronaut out of the space craft and refuses to let him back in. You see, Hal had made a mistake and could not admit it. How very human-like.

before electric typewriters and computers. Since I could type, buying my IIe let me explore the world of computing. It was great fun and allowed me to explore simple basic programing, even writing a program for the interpretation of blood gas test results. Within a short time, professional programmers were producing much more sophisticated versions. My skills were in the medical, not the computer field. I need not burden you with the progress in the computer world.

As my medical practice matured, my use of computers kept up with their ability to make life easier. My specialty practice needed quality reports to keep its referring physicians informed, as did my work interpreting hospital studies. The computers of the 90s and since allow for the creation of these. More ominously, the financial aspects of medical practices began to require computerization. Progress in technology and increased control over fees and payments by outside businesses and government required more and more computerization. Then, a little more than a decade ago, the electronic medical record appeared. It first was a way to organize the doctor's medical files, but integration with the financial aspects of practice rapidly followed. The electric, digital medical record was born. Hospital and medical practices, with significant government encouragement, widely adopted the electronic system. Use became mandatory for some.

> "*Open the pod bay doors, Hal,*" requested astronaut Dave Bowman.
>
> "*I'm sorry, Dave. I'm afraid I can't do that,*" responded Hal, the 9000 Computer.

"The X system does not allow that. I think you can work around it. You will need to go to the 'order' tab, then the 'misc' tab. That will get the dropdown menu for other items. It is probably listed there," the support staff cheerily reviewed for me. Their acceptance of the complexities of the digital medical record is probably based upon their knowledge of its inner working. Most of the staff were born after my IIe was manufactured. Raised with and around computers, their acceptance of these difficulties is as understandable as it is disturbing. Though their follow-up comment indicates dependency on a higher authority: "Sharon, Medical Record X's representative, can probably help us with that. I will reach out to her. I can have something for you in a few days." This interaction has become more and more common when a doctor working for a large group or organization runs into issues with documenting, placing orders, or communicating with their patients.

Don't misunderstand me. They are trying to be helpful. They definitely know more about the X electronic medical record than the physicians do. What is irritating is their acceptance that it is the holy grail of records. Their entire lives have been during the computer age. It leads them to accept all its faults and, I suspect, to not fully understand why just a few more clicks to memorize and perform does not leave me happy. What happens when the business Medical Record X changes the clicks, deletes the item or task needed, or I forget the clicks? I am back to square one.

> "*Dave, this conversation can serve no purpose anymore. Goodbye,*" concludes Hal when it tires of discussing opening the

> pod bay doors with Dave. Hal has made a decision, and it will not change. Dave will be left in space. Dave, using human ingenuity, ultimately finds an alternate way back into the space craft.

Recently it was announced, company X had added an upgrade that some of the support staff were using. It is a program to change a prepared patient message to a calmer, more comforting tone and words. We were told it has helped improve the patient's perception of a few of the staff messages where it has been used. How does it work? A message is prepared. You ask the program to review it. It does, and then it changes how the message is phrased and addressed to the patient. Red flags flew in my head. Is this the first step in eliminating the human contact in medical care? For example, just feed the result of a test into the system and it prepares and sends the message. Will it become similar to the multitude of robo calls, messages, and commercial computer chats to which we are now exposed? Yes, I am being a bit paranoid. At the least, it does indicate some of the support staff need to improve their communication skills.

> "*Just what do you think you're doing, Dave?*" Hal asks.
>
> "*Dave, stop. Stop, will you? Stop, Dave. Will you stop, Dave? Stop. Dave.*" Hal attempting to stop Dave from deactivating it.
>
> Hal's finial vocalizations: "*I'm afraid. I'm afraid. Dave. Dave, my mind is going. I can feel it. I can feel it. My mind is going.*"

Dave completed his mission without Hal. Following Dave's guidance, maybe we need to disable X. No, that would be like doing away with the car, a terrible thought. Without the automobile, modern society would crumble. There are cars made to go 180 miles per hour and travel through deserts and mountains with ruts for roads, but few will purchase them and even fewer will use those features. Unfortunately, the typical electronic medical record system comes with the 180 mile per hour and off-road options. Unlike the car of your choice, you are more a passenger than the driver of the record.

Those options on the electronic record are controls that constrain the medical practice to conform to insurance and government standards. We should recognize the dangers of its controlling nature. It is very similar to government. Governments have an essential role in allowing a free society to flourish, and too much government results in tyrannical control. In our era, China, North Korea, Cuba, and Russia are good examples of too much control. The computer has an important, almost essential role in medicine, but when controlled by self-interested parties, it can become tyrannical.

As the ultimate users, doctors, and maybe patients, need to police the features included in the computerization of the medical record. Let's not buy those controlling features. Remember, your role in most systems will be that of passenger, not driver, and it is going to be a long, frustrating, expensive ride.

Titles

There used to be a time when we wore our occupations proudly. I guess that is still the case, but the labels are not as clear anymore. Perhaps I just haven't learned to understand what they mean, or maybe I am just old-fashioned.

Recently, at a school reunion, an acquaintance bragged about the success of another school chum working in "healthcare." Upon questioning, I found the work was as an administrator for an insurance firm's HMO.

Later as I sat with several others, a casual comment struck me. Someone noted, "Well, all of the healthcare workers are sitting together." This group included the HMO executive, a medical office employee, a chiropractor, and a physician. It dawned on me that the term "healthcare worker" could define that group and a thousand other groups.

As a physician, I want to keep my patients well and work toward that goal. However, I care for the ill, not the healthy. The label "healthcare" worker doesn't sit well with me. I have worked hard for my professional standing. When I am asked what I do, I call myself a physician, but my announcement is often followed by the response, "So, you are a doctor?"

The title "Doctor" seems to carry its own definition for many people who have not worked in the medical field. No doubt it comes from prior physician contacts, personally or with family members, movies, television, and literature. The definitions often unrealistically represent a combination of Marcus Welby, Albert Schweitzer, and Michael DeBakey.

Like the term "healthcare," for which each speaker has his own definition and which is used too generously, the title "Doctor" creates an image.

The title implies more than just a degree. It implies an awareness, an experience, an evolution into human beings with unique roles and unique responsibilities; individuals who frequently face life, death, sorrow, grief, and joy; who experienced routinely what most only experience with catastrophic, life-defining events.

The title "Doctor" implies all of those things.

As physicians, I think we allow those trained in the profession to spend and spread our mystique too generously. Someone has a medical degree, and is therefore a doctor. The title implies that the individual cares for patients and is a physician or surgeon. We know that may not be the case.

Maybe we, those who practice or have mastered the art, should adopt a different term for the life we lead. Physician, surgeon—these words communicate the uniqueness of our profession. They represent who we are and what we do, a uniqueness over and above our training and degree. Maybe there needs to be a campaign to define physician and surgeon in order to alert the public to the hangers-on.

Hangers-on? Yes, we have those. They are our colleagues who have made the academic climb with us into our profession, but who have dropped out before practicing and mastering the art. Maybe they just finished school, internship, or residency. Maybe they went into a field that does not have traditional medical responsibilities.

We all enjoy the title "Doctor." It implies that we are a part of that fraternity of knowledge, the Hippocratic tradition, the Osler Way, the sense of being a physician, of being more than knowledgeable about disease and pathophysiology, of being a practitioner of the art of medicine. But should those who have left the fold before attaining that sense of responsibility continue to carry the title and what it implies?

They use the title "Doctor" to help them with business, insurance, hospital, university, or other work. Many doctors in those fields were and are physicians, surgeons, and clinicians. Most of them have earned the respect that the title "Doctor" or physician or surgeon commands. Unfortunately, some have not.

On their climb to success these businessmen, educators, and administrators with medical degrees often have not had the opportunity for that singular responsibility of patient care, including an ill patient who may die if you omit, forget, or neglect something in their care.

Why should I be concerned about those doctors, about labels, or about titles? They have lost their opportunities to be physicians or surgeons, to share the awesome responsibility of life and death and the opportunities to live the adventure of being physicians.

I understand why they would be proud of the title. But I am concerned when the title allows them to influence patient care, to manage patient care, to ration patient care, and to give reassurance to non-professionals that a knowledgeable, experienced clinician has reviewed patient care decisions and policies.

At a recent meeting, I had lunch with a young M.D. who was pursuing a career in administration. Following residency training, he began serving as a medical director for an insurance plan. As he spoke, it became clear why he had chosen that career path.

He listed his reasons for the decision, including lifestyle, income, leadership opportunities, and being part of the big picture, but as he spoke he communicated more. He communicated his dislike of ill people, his frustrations with trying to care for them, his inability to understand why they did not follow his directions, and his contempt for their questioning his authority as their doctor.

Here was someone doing a job with an insurance plan that had to be done, needed to be done, and could only be done by a physician. While his degree said he was a doctor, he had never held the responsibilities and could not perform as a physician. Ironically, unable to cope with the individual patient, he had advanced to overseeing the care of many.

Since "Doctor" implies more than is real, I suspect the label "healthcare worker" implies some knowledge or special mystique that physicians, surgeons, and nurses used to have for themselves.

"Healthcare workers." Well, I guess the label may be a badge of honor to some. Those who support our efforts to care for the ill wish to share in our magic. Many fields do not have the role recognition that physicians, surgeons, and nurses enjoy.

They have my permission, for I know that they, more than others, recognize the wonders of being a physician. We tread a path they wish they could share.

The Business of Medicine

The business of medicine is complicated. It may not seem so to those who are only receiving care, but the processes and issues behind the scenes are very complex. It is similar to eating at a restaurant where the meal is served effortlessly and the food is perfect, but the meal's preparation and delivery require knowledge, skill, planning, and performance. Medicine is no different. It is just that more knowledge, planning, and effort are required to have a desired outcome, and the number of rules and regulations for those efforts are staggering. Along my path of becoming a physician, my reflections on medicine as a business have raised these thoughts and considerations.

Is the business of medicine the doctor's business? Yes and no. Within the business of medicine, there are countless types of personnel, facilities, suppliers, regulatory bodies, bill payors, and business structures. Each has an effect on the perceived and real quality of service and care, such as the available services and the cost of that care. In the American economic system, a mixture of independent, pseudo-independent, and government entities participates. There are regulations propagated by independent businesses and organizations, local and state governments, and the federal government that impact all of the entities and individuals involved. What and who are involved with the business of medicine? Let's look at some of the elements by reviewing a sampling of each:

Types of personnel

There are the doctors, of course. Advanced providers, such as nurse practitioners and physicians' assistants, are growing in numbers. There are nurses, assistants, secretaries, administrators, technicians, and other support people for the facilities and equipment being used. Many of these are required just for an office to function. Hospitals and other care facilities require all the above staff and more. The insurance companies, payment companies, and government programs have multiple levels of employees. They include those performing basic functions as well as administrators, doctors, and also chief executive officers, shareholders, and boards of trustees. The types and number of people involved are enormous.

Types of facilities

These include offices, clinics, diagnostic laboratories, sleep centers, radiographic facilities, urgent care facilities, hospitals, post-hospital extended care, nursing homes, pharmacies, durable medical equipment companies, and a variety of others.

Types of supplies

All of the supplies needed to run a home or hotel are also required in medical facilities. Medical equipment from tongue blades to computer tomographic scanners to surgical suites is needed. This is an amazingly long list including computers and computer support; water, electricity, and other utilities; and special diagnostic, laboratory, and therapeutic equipment and the supplies needed for their operation. There are thousands of supplies and suppliers. This list would include the businesses that support the personnel, such as accountants, lawyers, insurance companies, investment firms, and others. On the payment side, there are firms that manage insurance payments serving as clearing houses for money transfers. Pharmacies and the drug industry (manufacturers, developers, and suppliers) should be included on this list.

Types of regulatory bodies

Local business licenses and tax permits, as well as state licenses and permits, are just the beginning. The providers and personnel will need individual licenses appropriate for their training. There are national accrediting organizations for individuals, diagnostic facilities, hospitals, extended care facilities, and for almost every aspect of medical care. There are insurance plans that regulate the care of their enrollees by requiring memberships and accreditations, as well as government programs that require registration and regular updating. The list is extensive.

Types of payors

Some individuals still pay for healthcare with cash. Most participate in some form of insurance paid for by their employers, the government, or themselves. The insurance regulates the charges and pays all or a portion of them. Government plans have enrollees, set charges for any services provided to them, and pay those charges.

Types of business involved

There are single-owner businesses owned by physicians and other types of providers. Multi-person partnerships, professional corporations, limited liability companies, for-profit and not-for-profit corporations are all ownerships utilized by health-related companies.

Types of ownership

Physicians and other providers represent a small portion of ownerships, while communities, cities, states, and the federal government represent a much larger percentage. The majority of non-government ownerships are by nonmedical, non-healthcare individuals. These private nonmedical parties and the federal government are the main owners of the healthcare business. The corporations can be made up of a few owners or a multitude, with the largest companies listed on the stock exchanges. Yes, if you have a retirement plan, stock ownership, or employee investment plan, you probably are an owner of some portion of the business of medicine. The corporations often own other corporations that are running businesses in related fields. An example of this would be a health insurance company owning a corporation that operates hospitals.

Goals of ownership

Making a living is the goal of most of the personnel in healthcare. Most would like a good living, and some, a great living. Governments are involved to provide a service to their populations. Individuals invest in the businesses providing healthcare and the services and products needed to make a profit.

Doctors and Physicians play a central role in the care of patients. However, they play a minor role in the business of medicine and its cost. In America, the price of healthcare is indirectly controlled by the prices paid by the government for Medicare services. The payors set their contracted reimbursements to doctors and hospitals based upon the rates paid by the government through Medicare. Large medical groups composed of many doctors have some influence by being able to have non-medical, business-trained personnel help them navigate the complexities of the medical business world. Individual providers do not and are at a disadvantage.

Health-related businesses like health insurance companies and drug manufacturers are frequently massive in size. Health insurance companies may employ doctors for patient care, own hospitals and some of their suppliers, and have some ownership of drug manufacturers. These steps are to control costs and improve corporate profits, usually quite successfully, if judged by their stock prices and evaluations. Drug manufacturers work to produce breakthrough drugs that have high profit potential. They have a major influence with media through their advertising, with medical journals through their multi-million-dollar research publications, and with their major congressional lobbying efforts.

Patients have essentially no influence. Most of their expenses are hidden from them and paid by their employer or possibly a government plan. Some may pay with cash or pay for their own insurance, but they are in the minority.

A doctor's influence is also limited. Most doctors are unable to negotiate prices because of their small business size, although some elite subspecialities may be an exception to that statement. Reimbursements for doctors are at the whim of the insurance companies' contract rates. Some rates are so low the doctor has to reduce the time for each patient and see more patients each day just to meet the expenses of the practice.

It is obvious to me that the conundrum of the business of medicine is beyond the scope of anyone's control. Like civilized life itself, it is complicated. America has benefited from our capitalistic economic system, as has medical care. But medical care is becoming more and more out of reach of the citizen. In our civilized life, the markets are full of objects for those citizens who can purchase what they need and want. Medicine is already a semi-socialized system, and the cost is growing. Citizens cannot purchase what they want. It is controlled or not available. Americans do not have a single intermediary (insurance) deciding which tomato they will buy and at what store. In medicine, they do.

In the business of medicine, there is a need for limitations. There should be guardrails on the system. A free market system with those guardrails will result in healthier citizens and less costly medical care.

The current concept is to encourage competition between large corporations. Often, these corporations will be vertically monopolistic (owning insurance companies and hospitals while employing their own doctors and clinic staffs). They can be horizontally monopolistic (owning all the hospitals in a region or being the predominant insurance company in a region). Maybe in healthcare, corporations should be limited to their field of origin (insurance, medications, etc.). Maybe the for-profit healthcare businesses should not be allowed to be monopolies. Maybe corporations organized to be profit-making ventures for their shareholders should not be allowed ownership of medical practices, groups, hospitals, or other care facilities.

Maybe the patient should be the owner of any medical insurance policy no matter who pays for it. Maybe that policy should continue to be in force as long as it is paid for and not tied to employment. Maybe health insurance and health expenses should be treated the same under tax laws no matter who purchases and pays for them.

Physicians and doctors may be minor players in the business of medicine, but they should understand the business and its complexities. They should work toward influencing those they interact with to help convince them of the need for appropriate guidelines and less control. What does your doctor think about the business of medicine? You should ask.

Defining a Physician

SECTION THREE

Defining a Physician –

INTRODUCTION TO SECTION THREE

In life, there are few endeavors that produce such a sense of accomplishment as being a Physician. Dealing with humans in need and providing educated care and direction makes it one of the most rewarding callings in life. And if a doctor is fortunate enough to participate in expanding to any degree the scope of medical knowledge, the personal rewards are even greater. My reflections have led me to consider what, beyond the title "doctor," makes a Physician. What are the differences? Are there special attributes a doctor needs to have or to learn? This section describes my perception of those differences and relates some of the characteristics and requirements, such as education, experience, integrity, and inner strength, that make up a physician.

Multiple features characterize a Physician. Many are personal, but medicine is far from just personal attributes. The Physician's work is heavily influenced by society, government, professional organizations, schooling, pharmaceutical companies, mentors, professional colleagues, medical journals, and medical trends. Those interests work to control or influence the doctor's attitudes and opinions. They can work alone or may collaborate or compete with each other. Sophisticated marketing, educational events, scientific arguments, rules, regulations, insurance requirements, and payment limitations are used to promote their interests. A true Physician's behavior, however, is mostly, as it should be, independent of these influences, being guided more by personal values and character.

Education matters. During medical school, students learn facts that teach them the general frameworks of health and disease, forming the basis of their medical knowledge for their careers. More specialized knowledge is acquired with postgraduate training as a resident doctor. In addition, the skills of locating and analyzing details about specific topics are acquired. Training is just the beginning. Physicians must watch for and seek newer facts that increase or change their basic knowledge. Medicine is in constant change. Being a Physician means life-long learning, study, and striving to follow and understand these changes. Are they real? Are they proven? How does the new information change what they do? How does new information compare with their past experiences? This is a daunting task and a skill that develops gradually.

There is a wide spectrum of individuals who choose to become Physicians: some are brilliant, most are intelligent, and many are diligent scholars. All discover soon upon entering training that the scope of information about illness and its diagnosis and treatment is enormous: far more vast than anyone, even the brilliant, can acquire and assimilate. They learn to organize the information and maintain a knowledge of the general aspects of all medicine. Most importantly, Physicians need to recognize what they do not know and how to easily retrieve that information when it is needed in their work. It is the enormity of the body of medical knowledge that has led to specialized fields of study and care in medicine.

Physicians' attitudes toward the profession and toward their patients are developed and adopted somewhat during training, but these are traits that individuals will have established to a large extent before entering medical school. They will reflect the personalities, the beliefs, and the culture of youth. A person's strengths and beliefs of character upon entering medical training will determine the effects of that training on their attitudes as a professional. Over the next thirty or more years, the doctor's work will be a demonstration of those attitudes. Some attitudes and behaviors are, or should be, common to all Physicians.

The Hippocratic Oath, the ancient oath of healers, is still used by most Western medical schools. It lists the duties and obligations of a Physician and ought to be looked upon as a minimum standard by which a Physician should carry out those responsibilities. It should be a shared value of all those practicing medicine. But an education and an oath are not enough to produce the Physician one would choose to care for oneself or one's family. More is needed.

A practicing Physician meets and cares for all manner of individuals: rich and poor, intelligent and simple, clean and unwashed, as well as the other extremes of human beings, their behaviors, and personalities. All types will find their way to the Physician's care. A person entering the medical field or being trained as a doctor should have experienced as much of the spectrum of humanity as possible. Such experience allows for a better understanding of their patients and their ills. It leads to tolerance, acceptance, and empathy.

Finally, it may come as a surprise, but a Physician needs to be strong of mind, will, attitude, and body to meet the life they will experience. There will be financial strains, professional disagreements, practice arguments, long hours of work, unhappy patients, and legal strains. Life as a Physician is demanding and not for the faint of heart.

Living up to the ideals of being a Physician is one of life's highest goals. Becoming a Physician means striving to achieve those ideals. The honor of being a Physician is earned by pursuing and following them.

A Doctor? No, a Physician

Many trained to be a Doctor of Medicine seem to lack certain skills; perhaps they were not taught them or did not have them demonstrated. During my training years, I recall that limited portions of those skills were intermittently related to me by various Physicians, some taught, others just observed. Now, being far removed from the teaching of young doctors, I am unsure of their training in these skills. Interacting with some young doctors leads me to conclude not much has changed. The skills I am referring to would best be described as the "art of medicine," the skills demonstrated by seasoned Physicians caring for their patients.

I am treading on unsteady ground. A word's definition is not any one person's choice. Oh, yes, we each have our own idea of what a word means, our definition, but my concern is with the formal definition. The formal definition establishes what our language and culture perceive as a word's definition. What are the formal definitions of the words "doctor" and "physician"? And how do these compare and contrast with what I am attempting to define as a Physician? The formal definitions are briefly summarized below. My opinion will not influence these definers of the English language, but I believe my perception is more appropriate.

For *doctor* when referring to a person:

Merriam-Webster:

An eminent theologian, learned teacher, a person who has earned one of the highest academic degrees (such as a PhD) conferred by a university or a person awarded an honorary doctorate degree by a college or university. A person skilled or specializing in the healing arts.

Cambridge Dictionary:

A person with a medical degree whose job is to treat people who are ill or hurt. A person who has the highest degree (=qualification) from a college or university.

Collins:

Someone who is qualified in medicine and treats people who are ill. A dentist or veterinarian can be called doctor. Someone awarded the highest academic or honorary degree by a university.

For *physician*:

Merriam-Webster:

A person trained in the art of healing.

Cambridge Dictionary:

A medical doctor, especially one who has general skill and is not a surgeon.

Collins:

A person who is legally qualified to practice medicine; doctor of medicine. A person engaged in general medical practice, as distinguished from one specializing in surgery. A person who is skilled in the art of healing.

A review of these definitions certainly does not, in my view, give a clear picture of physicians or doctors, what they are, or how they may differ.

A university grants the degree of Doctor of Medicine to those who complete the required course of instruction in the basic fields of medicine. Being a Doctor of Medicine does not make one a Physician. Additionally, many achieve the high academic designation of doctor who are trained in nonmedical fields. Those who receive the degree can and should use their title "Doctor" proudly.

So, what is my problem? Are the definitions inappropriate or unsuitable? I think insufficient is a better description. Over my decades of medical practice, I have noted differences in how individual doctors carry out the clinical practice of medicine. Some are good and some not so good. An added ingredient makes good doctors, or skilled doctors. It makes them what Merriam-Webster means in its definition of a physician: "skilled in the art of healing." That is the essence of being a Physician.

You may wonder how I became interested in the definitions of doctors and physicians. It started many decades ago. During my medical school training, the last year had a required period when students spent time with a primary care doctor. Most of these doctors were in small rural towns. My assignment in western Oklahoma was in a town of about three thousand souls with three primary care doctors. I learned a great deal during those weeks. First, I felt that I was probably not smart enough to become or remain up to date in such a broad field. It actually made me look toward specializing. My second realization was that they were very good at their jobs, much more professional in many ways than the doctors

I was exposed to at the medical center. I did not realize it at the time, but they were Physicians.

Later in my training and before I decided on my future line of study, I learned more about the differences between Physicians and doctors. I was in training at the university hospital and assigned for a period of time with the pulmonary disease service (lung specialists). It was on the traditional hospital rounds that a difference struck me. The individuals on rounds included the senior staff attending doctor, one or two doctors training in the specialty (pulmonary fellows), medical residents (general internal medicine trainees, of which I was one) and interns (doctors in the first year of training after graduation with the Doctor of Medicine degree). It was quite a group to come into a hospital room to help with the patient's care. The pulmonary rounds traditionally started in the x-ray department, where each patient's x-rays were reviewed and the patient's history was presented by the pulmonary fellow. Afterward, we would then proceed to the hospital floors where the individual patients were visited.

The attending staff doctor was a nationally known individual whose textbook on the field was published shortly after my time on the service. He was scholarly, sophisticated, composed, professional, and imposing. The patient was a rancher from western Oklahoma. The patient's significant stature, along with his chiseled, creased, and darkly tanned face, would have made him an instant cowboy star in Hollywood. I had spoken with him earlier. His voice and conversation reinforced the image of a rough cowboy. His responses were direct, short, and to the point.

The attending doctor was introduced to the "cowboy." It was almost like magic. In a few minutes, they were chatting as if they had known each other since childhood. In those few minutes, the attending had earned the patient's trust and created a bond. Later, in the hall, the attending reviewed the information he had obtained about the patient's illness. It was far more than the junior doctors, including me, had obtained. I was struck by the attending's skill. During my time on that service, I observed the attending was almost always able to bond and communicate with the patient. The patients were not in awe of his reputation or stature in the medical world. They were unaware of it. They were aware that he seemed to understand what they needed and the questions they had: What is wrong? What needs to be done? What are the next steps? What effect will it have on my life? These he anticipated, answered, or helped them understand. He seemed to know what they were thinking. His calm, thoughtful, relaxed approach seemed to reassure them. He was empathetic of their situation. He treated them as human beings, almost as family, not just as patients. At the time I did not realize it, but what I witnessed was a skilled Physician relating to a patient. The attending was one good doctor! He truly was a Physician!

Most Doctors of Medicine do not meet my definition of a Physician. They do not have the knowledge, skills, communication ability, or persona that is required. Patient care is a demanding task, and mastering it begins early in our training. The ability of an individual to relate to another can be learned, but it is largely formed by our personality and experiences we develop before maturity. The often-stressful interaction of doctor and patient requires a calm, confident doctor: one comfortable with his knowledge and skills that are developed with time and experience. But the basic enjoyment of people and connecting to them is often developed at home and carried throughout our lives. Interacting with patients and making them comfortable is a task so daunting that many of those in training look for alternative ways to use their degree to participate in medicine. They try to distance their work from that patient interaction.

Doctors can specialize to free themselves from the ongoing responsibilities of patient care or significant direct patient contact by focusing on one aspect of medicine or working in a non-patient-care area. A Doctor of Medicine can specialize in certain fields, such as heart, lung, kidneys, stomach, brain, or skin. They can specialize in certain procedures, including surgery, radiology, or laboratory medicine. They can even specialize in physical locations, such as emergency medicine, hospitalist, or intensive care. A whole different world of work awaits the willing doctor in academic medicine, hospital administration, business, insurance, and government work. Work as a healer, however, is not performed in many fields of endeavor that a Doctor of Medicine may choose. Without a doubt, they, like nonmedical doctors, should proudly use the title of Doctor that they have earned. However, it is the doctor interacting with patients who may become a Physician.

The universities and hospitals that are training the future Doctors of Medicine influence and model medical practice for them, but they often do not provide that extra skill set, training their Doctor of Medicine graduates to be Physicians. Increasingly, students are chosen by these institutions for their potential benefit to the institutions where they train and to the profession of academic medicine, to be the future scientists, teachers, and leaders of the medical world. They need to be brighter, smarter, and greater achievers than others. The requirements leave less time before entering medical school to experience life other than their world as a student, less time to mature as an adult. They want to train doctors who will excel in the medical schools' work. That work is groomed into the students. It is the medical care provided by large clinics: teaching, performing research, and taking care of complex, unusual, and demanding medical issues. Those are all noble goals and skills, but most patients receive their care through individual doctors and small clinics, where little, if any, research and teaching is carried out. A Doctor of Medicine, at a minimum, should be competent as a foot soldier in the war against human disease.

When I trained those decades ago, the unspoken communication was that only those who were not going to excel went into the direct patient care fields. Yet that is where most care takes place and where most doctors will work. I do not think that has changed. Interestingly, it is where I spent most of my working career.

A doctor's practice location and field of work have an effect on the extent of his patient care work. A smaller or rural community will require more patient care responsibilities. A specialist in a large medical group, university, or hospital can shift those responsibilities to doctors in primary care and doctors in training. The same specialist in a less urban environment will have more patient care responsibilities. Procedure, testing, and location specialists (surgeons, radiologists, or emergency room doctors) will have different exposures but still have direct patient interactions. Their exposure to direct patient interactions will depend upon their specialty and responsibilities. The selection of a specialty can limit exposure to patients to a single visit or none at all. The Physician will demonstrate the same skills with those patient interactions, be they frequent and repeated or one time only for a brief period. It is the quality of the interaction that a Physician provides, not its frequency or duration.

Who, then, is a doctor? My definition: A Doctor of Medicine is a person who has been trained in medical science and granted by a training institution a degree certifying his training. A doctor may work in many fields, including both patient care and non-patient-care situations

Who, then, is a Physician? That is a much more complex question. It is what all practicing Doctors of Medicine should want to be. Foremost, a Physician is most often involved in the direct medical care of patients. It is not the field of work nor the time spent in direct patient care that determines a Physician. It is the skill of interacting with the patient, respecting the oath of our profession, and maintaining the knowledge needed that constitute the Physician. In my view, a Doctor of Medicine is not a Physician based upon his field of work, training, certifications, or honors. He is a Physician based on his personal and practice characteristics and behaviors.

Trained in the science of medicine, the Physician listens, assesses, describes, recommends, assists with decisions, and directs testing and therapy with follow-up care for his patients. The Physician is empathetic and communicates well with all manner of patients from all walks of life. The Physician may have strong views on political, religious, and social issues that guide their personal behavior, but when performing their medical role, they conceal them behind the Physician's mask.

A Physician recognizes his responsibilities for patients under his care. He is working for the patient, not the clinic, hospital, or insurance company. There is a link of responsibility. When we are ill, a Physician is that Doctor of Medicine that we want to care for us.

A Physician is skilled in the art of healing.

A Doctor's Oath

When do the traditions, the mantle of being a healer, begin? In our Western system, the oath of the healer, the Hippocratic Oath, is given to those who graduate with the degree of Doctor of Medicine. For most, it is part of the graduation ceremony. Is graduation an appropriate time? Is the Oath appropriate for all those who receive the degree? Why are there calls for changes in the Oath?

Medical school is difficult. The student is under pressure to learn, memorize, communicate, perform, and complete tasks at a high level. All the while, the student is exposed to the good and bad of human behavior along with the macabre and the diseases that await us all. Sensitivities of sight, smell, and touch are stressed by being insulted to the extreme. Time becomes a blur as long hours, nights of duty, reports, and exams each pile one upon another, overlapping, and only ending at graduation. The stress is physical and mental. By graduation, the student has changed and is also eager to finish the process and graduate.

Each person encounters both a shared and a unique set of experiences as they travel though the process. Upon receiving the Doctor of Medicine degree, their careers will diverge even further. Graduation is the last time when most of those experiences are shared—the last time before the new Doctors of Medicine's career paths diverge. It is at graduation when the Hippocratic Oath is pledged, placed on one of the pinnacle points in their career paths. The Oath's significance and seriousness is lost as it seems to take a minor role in the ceremony. It is like asking a medal-winning Olympic athlete to swear to train and live like an Olympian after winning the race. Their minds could not be further from the deeper meaning of the Oath. They have crossed the finish line, the first of many in their careers.

Is there a better time or place in the training of the healer to state those obligations? Is there a reason for not repeating the oath of responsibilities as their career progresses? Should everyone graduating with that Doctor of Medicine degree take an oath meant for those who will work with patients and perform as healers? All are reasonable questions to ask.

In Western societies, those with a Doctor of Medicine degree have many possible career paths. Most begin with medical apprenticeships that the profession terms "residencies." There are some who bypass these traditional professional pathways and proceed directly into alternate paths such as administration, research, or entrepreneurial endeavors. Both groups, the traditional and non-traditional, have reason, I believe, to take the Oath. Career paths change often. It seems appropriate for those graduating to make the moral commitments to our profession. They have been prepared to enter the profession, even though not all will do so.

Those shared experiences of a clinical nature, occurring early in a medical student's career, need to be carried out in the context of our medical ethics and education. Students would benefit from reciting and reviewing the Oath as their years of training progress. My limited exposure to recent or current students is encouraging. I have been told of one school where the Oath is emphasized early and often in each student's training. Another student's school gives limited emphasis to the Oath, as mine did decades earlier. The standard of waiting until the student graduates to have them commit to the Oath seems to minimize its importance as the benchmark for the behaviors and practices of Doctors of Medicine.

Does taking the Oath make a Doctor of Medicine a Physician? No, of course not, but it does lay the foundation as to what is expected of those heading into the world as a Doctor of Medicine.

What is the Hippocratic Oath? Why is it important? For over a century, it has been a tradition of schools teaching Western medicine in the United States and Europe that the students take the Oath. For many schools, the tradition spans several centuries.

The Oath is thought to have originated in ancient Greece and has been ascribed to Hippocrates, but that is historical speculation. Hippocrates lived at the time of Socrates and Plato. He was well known in his own time and produced some seventy written compositions on medical subjects, which was a significant achievement, even by current standards. Of those, sixty have survived until modern times. Helen Askitopoulou and Antonio Vgontzas, medical and Hippocratic scholars, believe that these writings provided a great message: "that (*practicing*) medicine is a difficult but important art, inseparable from the highest morality and the love of humanity with emphasis on the individual patient and his illness."

In medieval times, the Oath was used in the Middle East, and it became of interest to Western scholars during the Renaissance. It is thought to have been written in approximately 400 BC, and its acceptance as an appropriate oath for newly trained doctors is clouded in history. By the last half of the twentieth century, it was commonly sworn at graduation ceremonies. The last few decades have seen increased concerns and complaints about its use, and many schools now modify some portions of the Oath.

It is interesting to observe older forms of the Oath. Easily available sources present several classic forms with variations in the wording. The forms change with a translator's choice of words. Some are found with a slightly different meaning or a shift in meaning that will often alter the perception of the Oath's purpose. The translators may be influenced by religious or cultural factors. The choices may be inconsequential, consequential, innocent, or purposeful. Scholars debate these issues, and medical school faculties modify the Oath for their students. For this discussion, it is of interest but would be a digression to more than superficially cover some of those issues. Of the oaths I reviewed, I have chosen the form presented by Askitopoulou and Vgontzas in which to highlight the words and subjects covered. This is an older or classic form of the Oath.

The Hippocratic Oath – A Classic Form[3]

> I swear by Apollo the physician, and Asclepius and by Health ['Hygeia'] and Panacea and by all the gods as well as goddesses, making them judges (*witnesses)*, to bring the following oath and written covenant ['sygrafi'] to fulfillment, in accordance with my power and my judgment;
>
> To regard him who has taught me this téchnē ['*art*'] as equal with my parents, and to share, in partnership, my livelihood with him and to give him a share

3 Italicized words appearing in parentheses were added by Askitopoulou and Vgontzas for clarity of the translation. With the exception of "art," words in brackets are the original Greek words that were translated. Italics, parentheses, square brackets, and quotation marks are all in the original Askitopoulou and Vgontzas text.

when he is in need of necessities, and to judge the offspring (*coming*) from him equal to (*my*) male siblings, and to teach them this téchnē, should they desire to learn (*it*), without fee and written covenant ['sygrafi'], and to give a share both of rules and of lectures, and of all the rest of learning, to my sons and to the (*sons*) of him who has taught me and to the pupils who have both made a written contract and sworn by a medical convention but by no other.

And I will use regimens for the benefit of the ill in accordance with my ability and my judgment. But from (*what is*) to their harm or injustice ['adikia'] I will keep (*them*).

And I will not give a drug that is deadly ['pharmakon thanassimon'] to anyone if asked (*for it*), nor will I suggest the way to such a counsel.

And likewise I will not give a woman a destructive pessary ['pesson fthorion'].

And in a pure and holy way I will guard my life and my téchnē.

I will not cut, and certainly not those suffering from stone, but I will cede (*this*) to men (*who are*) practitioners of this activity.

Into as many houses as I may enter, I will go for the benefit of the ill, while being far from all voluntary and destructive injustice ['adikia'], especially from sexual acts both upon women's bodies and upon men's, both of the free and of the slaves.

And about whatever I may see or hear in treatment,

> or even without treatment, in the life of human beings—things that should not ever be blurted out outside—I will remain silent, holding such things to be unutterable ['arreta'] (*sacred, not to be divulged*).
>
> If I render this oath fulfilled, and if I do not blur and confound it (*making it to no effect*) may it be (*granted*) to me to enjoy the benefits both of life and of téchnē, being held in good repute ['doxazomenos'] among all human beings for time eternal. If, however, I transgress and perjure myself, the opposite of these.

The Hippocratic Oath is rooted in swearing an oath to live up to standards for the profession of being a doctor. It asks the gods of the fifth century BC Greeks and all gods and goddesses to be witness to the Oath. Who are these gods? Much of the historical information is speculation.

> Apollo – A classical Greek god dating to before 700 BC. Legends tell of his ability to control health and illness. They also place him as the father of Asclepius.
>
> Asclepius – More than two thousand years ago, Asclepius was a Greco-Roman god of medicine. Thought to have been a skillful physician in Greece's early history, he was worshiped as a god by 600 to 500 BC. His father was considered to be Apollo.
>
> Hygeia – The Greek goddess of health, cleanliness, and hygiene. Her father was thought to be Apollo and her brother Asclepius and sister Panacea.
>
> Panacea – Greek goddess of universal remedies. Her father was thought to be Apollo and her brother Asclepius and sister Hygeia.

Hippocrates – A Greek physician of great standing who lived 460–375 BC. While the Hippocratic Oath bears his name, there is little evidence that he penned it. His reputation was one of high ethical and professional standards.

These ancient Greek gods of healing were worshiped and considered sacred, although now they are gods from history. An oath is a solemn, formal pledge by an individual that they will do what they are pledging. The Hippocratic Oath was meant to be just such a commitment.

The Oath can be viewed as a statement of ethics for the doctor to follow in the profession of medicine. I believe most, on reading it, would agree that the ethical standards are what should be expected of, and appropriate for, doctors and Physicians.

But times have changed, and efforts to change the Hippocratic Oath are ever present. We need to look at the Oath in a little more detail before we leave it.

The Hippocratic Oath

Through the centuries, the Hippocratic Oath has remained a subject of praise, ridicule, and debate. Despite that, it has been remarkable in its resilience, and it has remained widely accepted and used, although those calls for changes are still being voiced. Recently, I looked at the national medical database, PubMed, for articles reviewing the Hippocratic Oath. I found over one thousand published articles. Reviewing a few, I realized that most of the recent ones presented the Oath as being out of date and offered suggestions for change. A few called for eliminating the practice altogether.

Why do some want change? Are their concerns due to what the Oath promises? Is it a result of the varied manners in which "Doctors of Medicine" practice and are employed or because of political calls for changes in and paying for "healthcare"? These concerns led me to provide you with my thoughts about why changes are being suggested. This will not be an extensive review but enough to point out some of those issues.

An oath can be separated into the invocation (a call for witnesses to the taking of the oath), the pledges (promises, prohibitions, and commitments), and the consequences (the rewards and punishments) of observing or not observing those pledges. The promises, prohibitions, and commitments in the Hippocratic Oath form the core of all medical ethics. In my previous essay ("A Doctor's Oath"), I have introduced a classic form of the Hippocratic Oath. Let's look at it now in more detail.

The Invocation[4]

> I swear by Apollo the physician, and Asclepius and by Health ['Hygeia'] and Panacea and by all the gods as well as goddesses, making them judges (*witnesses*), to bring the following oath and written covenant ['sygrafi'] to fulfillment, in accordance with my power and my judgment;

The gods selected for mention were the gods of the ancient Greeks (2500 years old), not the god of Judaism (6,000–7,000 years old), Christianity (2000 years old), Islam (1400 years old), or the ancient Far Eastern religions. This is a difficult point for some and leads to a desire to change the Oath. Certainly, the monotheistic god of my Judeo-Christian upbringing does not fit well with this call to all gods and goddesses.

However, to a young man and now to a much older man, this part of the ancient Oath stresses the commitment to a higher authority. As scholars have pointed out, this is a request, an invocation to witness the oath taker, not a prayer to an ancient or foreign god. I am happy with that. We are taking an oath to be witnessed by our sacred beliefs, not those of ancient Greece. If an ancient Greek god happens to listen in, it would be so much the better.

With the current secular trends, lack of moral standards, atheism, and agnosticism, some would like to remove this type of reference altogether. I still think it is

4 Italicized words appearing in parentheses were added by Askitopoulou and Vgontzas for clarity of the translation. With the exception of "art," words in brackets are the original Greek words that were translated. Italics, parentheses, square brackets, and quotation marks are all in the original Askitopoulou and Vgontzas text.

an essential part of the Oath. Who would those individuals call to witness their oath, their lawyer or banker? This invocation has been changed and even deleted in many of the forms in current use.

The Oath is pledged to the Greek gods of healing and health. Is there any chance that their worship as gods could be based on real individuals from centuries or millennia earlier? We will never know. But just as the ancient Greeks called as a witness a higher authority that they recognized, we should ask the higher authority of our beliefs to be our witness.

The Pledges

Duties to the Profession

> To regard him who has taught me this téchnē (*'art'*) as equal with my parents, and to share, in partnership, my livelihood with him and to give him a share when he is in need of necessities, and to judge the offspring (*coming*) from him equal to (*my*) male siblings,

Equally with our parents, our educators should be honored. However, in twenty-five hundred years much has changed in the world of medical education. What was a craft and art learned as a gift from an individual now is a highly institutionalized process. The training is paid for by the student, the student's family, scholarships, and government institutions. Retired medical educators are not in need of support.

> and to teach them this téchnē, should they desire to learn (*it*), without fee and written covenant ['sygrafi'], and to give a share both of rules and of lectures, and of all the rest of learning, to my sons and to the (*sons*) of him who has taught me and to the pupils who have both made a written contract and sworn by a medical convention but by no other.

Those who pursue practicing medicine are fortunate. Medical doctors are perpetual teachers. If anything, they tend to teach too much. For those who have been accepted into medical education training, there is no shortage of practicing doctors willing to assist in that training. Most institutions have a large number of doctors who volunteer to teach medical students, residents, and associated medical personnel.

The Physician's Ethical Code

This portion of the Oath's pledges forms the core of medical ethics, behavior, and responsibilities that doctors are to follow.

The Promise to Benefit the Ill

> And I will use regimens for the benefit of the ill in accordance with my ability and my judgment. But from (*what is*) to their harm or injustice ['adikia'] I will keep (*them*).

This is what practicing doctors do or should do. This does not say the doctor will devise and order for the patient based on the latest insurance or government guidelines or the greater community's good. Often, suggested changes are directed toward public health or fashionable social issues, with fewer concerns for the care of the individual.

Despite general opinion to the contrary, the direct statement "Do no harm" does not appear in the Oath. It is from a much earlier Hippocratic document, *Epidemics I*. The portion "But from (*what is*) to their harm or injustice I will keep (*them*)" is stating the same principle.

The Prohibitions

> And I will not give a drug that is deadly ['pharmakon thanassimon'] to anyone if asked (*for it*), nor will I suggest the way to such a counsel.

The terminating of a human life is an extremely serious matter. The current lack of religious ethics along with secular indulgences and agnostic and atheistic beliefs have led to political and social upheavals regarding assisted suicide. Our ancient forebearers were firm on the issue. Modern doctors often support it and want this portion of the Oath removed. Assisted suicide has become a call of the progressives in our society and is even legally permitted in a few locations and countries. Doctors of Medicine participating in these practices are not keeping the Oath. I would not consider them healers and believe they should not practice medicine.

This portion of the Oath served as the source of medical ethics evidence used in the Nazi war crimes trial that led to the conviction of German doctors who had performed human experimentation on prisoners during World War II.

Many have interpreted this to mean "prohibit comfort care" for those near the end of life. Scholars differ on this. I agree with those who say this clause does not prohibit that care.

> And likewise I will not give a woman
> a destructive pessary ['pesson fthorion'].

This respected translation of the Oath has only this comment regarding abortion. It is important to note that in 400 BC in Greece, the words used were "pesson fthorion." It was at that time a specific physical device soaked in special fluids, not sterilized, and placed in the vagina to induce abortion. The use of such an unclean foreign body was considered very dangerous even two and a half millennia ago. It is the only comment in the early Greek forms of the Oath regarding abortions. Versions from the past several centuries may contain more prohibitive restrictions than those of the ancient Greeks, depending upon the interpretations and religious orientations.

Current debates about abortion are heated, opinionated, and, for the most part, uncompromising. Few practicing doctors have need to participate in these medical issues in their patient care work. For those who do, this can be a troubling portion of the Oath. This statement does not appear to prohibit abortion. The Oath taken by many medical graduates omits this section.

Commitment to Professional and Personal Integrity

> And in a pure and holy way I will guard my life and my téchnē.

This statement is a pledge to live life at a standard that all would respect. It is directing a doctor to live in an ethical manner, not with a condescending, arrogant, or egotistical view of others because of their standing in society. Unfortunately, self-reflection, tolerance, and ethical behavior are not found in all of those practicing medicine.

Recognizing Personal Limitations

> I will not cut, and certainly not those suffering from stone, but I will cede (*this*) to men (*who are*) practitioners of this activity.

In most developed civilizations, training in medicine precedes training in surgery. The statement limits the doctor to providing the care that he is trained to provide as the circumstances require. A Doctor of Medicine trained as a surgeon can be a Physician as much as a non-surgeon can. The stone referred to in this statement is thought to be bladder stones.

Care of the Patient, Benefit, and Prohibitions

> Into as many houses as I may enter, I will go for the benefit of the ill, while being far from all voluntary and destructive injustice ['adikia'], especially from sexual acts both upon women's bodies and upon men's, both of the free and of the slaves.

Doctors learn and are aware of many private details of the patient and the patient's family's lives. They deal with the patients when they are most vulnerable and weak. Patients and their families view their Physicians and doctors as special and have idealistic views of them. It would be more than improper for the doctor to use such information or weakness to their personal advantage.

Patient's Confidentiality Commitment

> And about whatever I may see or hear in treatment, or even without treatment, in the life of human beings—things that should not ever be blurted out outside—I will remain silent, holding such things to be unutterable ['arreta'] (*sacred, not to be divulged*).

This promise predated current privacy laws by 2,500 years. Doctors and Physicians recognized this as paramount in their care of patients. Current government and insurance requirements for non-professionals and businesses to have access to this information have made such legal restrictions a requirement.

Consequences

> If I render this oath fulfilled, and if I do not blur and confound it (*making it to no effect*) may it be (*granted*) to me to enjoy the benefits both of life and of téchnē, being held in good repute ['doxazomenos'] among all human beings for

> time eternal. If, however, I transgress and perjure myself, the opposite of these.

And so it should be.

Some academic doctors and others in non-care areas of work would like to add wording to the Oath stressing the doctor's responsibility to the community and its general health. Since the Oath focuses on the responsibilities of the doctor attending to patients under his care, I see no place for establishing community or broader responsibilities under this oath, especially since they may conflict with the care of the individual.

The Oath is amazing in its scope. Despite what academics and others say, it still to this day covers the care of a patient by the doctor. This ancient code of healers remains as pertinent today as it was 2,500 years ago. When the Oath is read in its ancient form, the immensity of its meaning seems clear. When considered, it means the doctor will have a certain set of values that will guide his professional life. Few are eligible to take it. Fewer still are able to live up to it. Those who do likely will deserve the title of Physician.

Physicians, Doctors and The Oath

If the Hippocratic Oath serves as a model for being a Physician, how does it contribute to defining the difference between a Doctor of Medicine and a Physician? Most Doctors of Medicine take the Oath. Taking the Oath and honoring it are two different activities, however. Honoring the Oath is what molds and provides the structure that allows doctors to become Physicians.

The Oath may serve as an excellent standard for the practice of medicine, but it is distant from a doctor's world. Maybe it is the place, the time, or the way that it is administered. Maybe it is the career a doctor chooses that makes it appear irrelevant. Maybe it is the demands of the business system required to practice medicine. Or maybe the doctors do not see it as a pledge of their personal honor and, as a consequence, forget it.

The timing of its administration plays a big role in its acceptance. Recall that it is the graduating Doctor of Medicine who takes the Oath. It is taken immediately before the degree is given, just after the graduate has satisfactorily completed four difficult years that include thousands of classwork hours, on-call nights at the teaching hospital, hours of study, and multiple examinations. The graduation is a formal affair. Most students view it as a necessary evil, even though families and friends enjoy the ceremony. The Hippocratic Oath traditionally has been a part of that ceremony. Some students are being introduced to and mentored in the Oath early in their schooling, but I doubt most students have more than a superficial knowledge of it and have read or even considered the Oath before that day. It is often taken in a perfunctory manner. It would be an unusual individual who would say, "I can't live up to that. Don't give me that degree." So the Oath is taken, usually for the only time in the Doctor of Medicine's career.

I believe there should be more commitment to the Oath and the ethics of our profession before the end of training. Maybe knowledge of the Oath, the pledges to be made, and the probable lifelong obligations it requires should be part of medical schools' acceptance reviews. It is reassuring that during student training some schools introduce the Oath at the side of a doctor before that first visit with a real patient. Maybe there should be repeated emphasis on the Oath throughout our careers. Since post-graduate training programs often do not have formal commencement ceremonies, organized medicine should consider sponsoring a Hippocratic Oath day each year for all to remember our pledge.

Choosing a perfect time to commit to the healing profession by taking an oath is difficult, if not impossible. With the multitude of career paths for those receiving the Doctor of Medicine degree, selecting an appropriate time is daunting and would vary for each career. We degree holders often change career paths as we age, and that adds to the confusion of selecting a different time to take an oath as a healer. I, for one, believe we should consider adding additional times to reaffirm our oath both before and after graduation with that Doctor of Medicine degree. It would increase the Physicians in our world.

In my maturity, I find it easy to suggest solutions, but it does seem that medical students should be exposed to the Oath early in their studies and on a regular basis in addition to the graduation ceremony. The pledges a Doctor of

Medicine is making apply to many of the students' activities as they interact with patients during training.

I would ask my incoming students to tell me their expectations for a career in medicine and what they know about the Oath. Would they be able to live up to such a commitment?

Why should the Oath not be reaffirmed? Oaths by their nature are often repeated; churches, organizations, and governments do so. The repetition helps those making the pledge to remind themselves of their promises and commitments. I believe it would be helpful if Doctors of Medicine reaffirmed their commitments on a regular basis.

A tradition could be encouraged for all those actively caring for patients—a yearly re-taking of the Hippocratic Oath. It would be a recurring reminder of those traits we pledged upon receiving that Doctor of Medicine degree and serve to restrain some undesirable tendencies that the mystique of being called Doctor often encourages. But I know there will be no national day. Doctor, pick your own day, and read the Oath.

What about differing career paths? There are many, and it is a major reason there probably will never be a national day to recognize and retake the Oath. Besides the role of assisting patients, there are administrators, government employees, entrepreneurs, and those in non-health-related fields who often do not have patient care responsibilities or work related to the medical profession. They may view the Oath as having little meaning for their work. I think it should hold meaning.

What about the multiple ways Doctors are paid? How do these affect the way we live out our Oath? The business of medicine is almost as complex as the study of medicine. Changes, even radical ones, occur frequently. Few work for the patient these days. Based on the work they do, Doctors of Medicine are paid differently. Solo practitioners and small groups of doctors are still usually paid based upon patient services. Larger groups, hospitals, universities, insurance companies, and health-related businesses pay their doctor employees differently. They are not paid based on patient services, but through salaries with benefits like paid protected time for teaching and research or bonuses for tasks completed. The greater the separation from patient care to corporate employee, the less the compensation is related to our Oath as healers and the more it is connected to the goals of the business. The greater the separation, the more likely the Oath will be disregarded. No matter how doctors are paid, the Oath should be the ethical foundation of their work. Unfortunately, the goals of health-related businesses often conflict with the roles of the providers of healthcare and certainly those of the practicing doctors. The doctors employed by many businesses are there to give the company the appearance of respecting the patient and patient care. Similar to the graduating doctors having to accept the Oath to get their degree, employed doctors work hard to perform well at their businesses. When these businesses start to cross the ethical lines of medicine, it is almost impossible for their doctors to stand against the will of the company as it could result in the loss of their business careers. Their commitment to the pledge of our ancient fellowship of healers will be broken, if it was ever intended to be kept.

Many Doctors of Medicine make no attempt to maintain a commitment to the code, as business success, recognitions, and even greed leads them away. It is hard to work outside of patient care as a Doctor of Medicine and remain committed to the promises made in the Oath. It is hard to work toward being wealthy and remain committed to those promises.

The doctor should regularly repeat the pledge, the Oath. Keep the pledge, and the doctor may become a Physician. It is an important first step. There will be no formal ceremonies. One day a doctor will realize that they have earned that title.

Healthcare Workers, Providers, Doctors and Physicians

Almost gone are the days of the solitary doctor meeting with patients in his home, his office, or their homes. Now, it is the doctor's office, the medical group's office, or the hospital's office. There is a reception room, a receptionist, and a medical assistant to direct you to your exam or consultation room. Once there, you will meet the director of your care (advanced provider, doctor, or physician) and a nurse to help with administering the recommended care. This book has been about my definition of a Physician and my experiences becoming one. It is about the characteristics that separate individuals with the same academic degrees who are doing the same work as well as the differences in their skills in the art of medicine. The care of the ill is a complicated business, with many people trained in a wide variety of fields. There are organizations, medical societies, academic associations, and colleges that contribute. There are many individuals and many different types of organizations that assist with providing the care and remedies needed for a patient to "live long and prosper." Most are not doctors. While focusing on what makes a Physician, it is important to consider those workers and organizations.

How do these individuals differ from medical doctors? The obvious differences include their education, their experiences during that education, their duration of study, their responsibilities, their degrees (of course), and ultimately the license granted by their government for their area of work. Note that I did not say intelligence. In my career, I have worked with many allied health and nursing individuals who were smart, bright, ethical, and as intelligent or more so than many Doctors of Medicine.

The education needed to work in medicine is determined by the chosen field. A role with fewer technical or learning requirements will have a shorter education and less practical experience exposure before graduates enter a working environment. The higher the requirements for knowledge and technical skills, the longer the education and practical experience time required for that role. Like the Doctor of Medicine, most of these individuals will face a professional lifetime of learning.

These jobs can be basic or may involve special skills, such as those of technicians in laboratories, radiology, surgery, and medicine. Nurses can have advanced training for special procedures, surgery, and caring for the critically ill. There are levels of their training that result in their legal ability to practice medicine with or independently of a medical doctor.

There are excellent programs that train individuals to become physician assistants. These individuals are not trained to be assistants to doctors, but are medical providers able to diagnose and treat medical conditions under the supervision of a licensed medical doctor. This requires a college bachelor's degree and advanced training for the role. The state will grant a license after qualifying exams are passed.

The nursing profession has increased its training from the basic level through the registered nurse designation to include master's degrees, doctorate degrees, and nurse practitioner certification. The nurse practitioner programs have lengthy training and demanding rigorous testing.

The different states have a variety of licensing levels for the highly trained nurse practitioners. The most restrictive licensing is similar to that of a physician assistant: the ability to work under the supervision of a licensed medical doctor. The most liberal states' laws allow an independent practice without supervision by a doctor, including ordering medical tests and prescribing medication.

Are they doctors? Some nurse practitioners have a doctorate in nursing. So, yes, they are doctors. Others? Many perform the work, most quite well, that traditionally has been the work of the Doctor of Medicine. But how do we address them? I'm not sure.

Do these medical providers have a code of ethics like the Hippocratic Oath for graduating doctors? Are they taught about the ethics of medical care? The answer is yes, but the presence of these practices is not clear to those of us far removed from their training and work. The nursing profession in the United States does use the Nightingale Pledge in a similar fashion. Created in 1893 and modeled on the Hippocratic Oath, it is now widely administered at nursing graduations. Canvassing several nurses and nurse practitioners in my acquaintances who span three decades in age, I found the Pledge, in their experiences, follows my experience with the Hippocratic Oath. After taking it at their graduations, they rarely encountered it again.

Physician assistants have an Oath that is taken at graduation in some institutions. I cannot assess the extent to which it is used in the training programs, and since my acquaintances in the field are extremely limited, I have no way to assess its role after graduation.

Initially, the reception of these advanced practitioners was varied. There were concerns by established doctors about the quality of the medical care they would provide.

Much of the original concern has dissipated. Many provide better and more complete care than some Doctors of Medicine. If my personal observations of the workings of advanced healthcare providers are of any value, they seem to tell me these advanced providers are often in many ways more grounded in the ethical aspects of their work than many doctors.

Unfortunately, many of these providers are abused and put in situations in which they have neither the knowledge nor the skills needed to perform. They are often hired by hospitals, clinics, and entrepreneurial doctors to do clinical work that may exceed their abilities. The employers or doctors may not be handy or available to assist them when needed. These employers and entrepreneurs may be in charge of many clinics, employing several advanced providers to staff them while they collect the fees for their work.

Problems can develop with these advanced providers (and with anyone providing healthcare, for that matter) if they do not recognize their limitations. They may feel they are as good as most medical doctors and may not have an internal ethical code. Sometimes they err in believing they know enough and do not need to ask for advice, while some may not have an available advisor to ask. Fortunately, this has not been common in my experience with them.

I hope these problems resolve. I believe that, as I have recommended for Doctors of Medicine elsewhere in this book, each type of healthcare worker and advanced provider would benefit from renewing their pledge or oath annually. In addition, clear labels or titles for the advanced providers should be established so they can be used consistently and properly.

In my opinion, the real differences between the various advanced-level providers and Doctors of Medicine are their training, their experiences, and the responsibilities carried within their roles. The facts learned are important, but they could be matched by any university that designed a program to do so. The experiences during the training that leads to a Doctor of Medicine degree are not so easily matched. Each individual's training, whether to be an advanced provider or a Doctor of Medicine, will differ. The training of most Doctors of Medicine will involve long hours of work under the supervision of practicing doctors, where, with time, one learns to become responsible for the patient's care. The student learns to cope, learns to understand, and begins to master the work a doctor is to do. Training to become a doctor includes learning to expect the unexpected and to know that it is the doctor's job to assess the situation. In a practice after training, the decisions begin and end with the doctor. A government license to practice medicine places significant responsibility on his shoulders. The doctors are often not alone when evaluating patients and making decisions. Nurses, technicians, and aides may be there to assist and share advice, but when the doctor is there, the ultimate decisions are the doctor's. These sometimes stressful experiences are what lead many Doctors of Medicine to leave the medical field, to seek work in non-patient-care areas, or to work in specialties with less direct care of patients. These experiences also make Doctors of Medicine different from other providers of care, who, while needing to make many difficult decisions on their own, may defer the decisions to a doctor.

Those who support doctors and physicians in their work do not receive the praise they are due. I believe there is a role for the Wizard here. Furthermore, like the Tin Man, Lion, and Scarecrow in the land of Oz, each character needs a fitting title for what they do. In the military, the responsibilities of a sergeant, captain, and colonel are evident to all. Healthcare providers need clear titles. Such titles should be recognized by all, but I doubt we will experience a general call for them. If I were King, I would give them appropriate titles and decree a day each year for them to review their oath or pledge.

Medical Societies, Associations and Colleges

I cannot leave this subject without making some comments on medical societies. It would be hoped that they would aid us in defining a Physician as opposed to just a doctor. All medical societies begin the same, develop in a similar fashion, and mature to be what they are. These organizations of doctors will use the terms society, college, and association as part of their names. There are steps in the development of these societies. Interestingly, the steps parallel the development of businesses. Businesses begin as startups, grow, and then mature. When mature, they maintain themselves, are taken over by other, usually larger businesses, or close. Do the societies help me in defining a Physician? Let us examine their role for doctors.

For several centuries, doctors have formed groups for many reasons. General organizations were formed based on geographic location. They proved useful for the doctors in their communities to share scientific and business information while providing social interactions with other doctors. In the United States, those groups of city, county, and state societies grew into the American Medical Association (organized in 1847), and it became the national voice for those state and local groups. Locally, these general organizations mostly retain the useful principles that led to their creations; however, the national organization has matured into a political machine representing a minority of practicing doctors.

In addition to these general organizations, there are specialty societies in most fields of medicine and surgery. Specialty societies began to develop over a century ago. There are general societies for adult medicine (the American College of Physicians, organized in 1915), surgery (the American College of Surgeons, organized in 1913), and children (the American College of Pediatrics, organized in 2002). As the practice of medicine developed and became more specialized, organizations of doctors for specific fields developed. Fields such as heart disease (American College of Cardiology, organized in 1947), kidney diseases (American Society of Nephrology, 1966), lung diseases (American Thoracic Society, 1905, and the American College of Chest Physicians, 1935), and skin diseases (American Academy of Dermatology Association, 1938) are examples of organ-specific medical organizations, while critical care medicine, emergency medicine, and hospitalist medicine are specialties that involve working in a specific location. In addition, there are organizations for doctors who specialize in certain procedures, such as those of the surgical specialists, the radiologists, and the anesthesiologists. The list of medical organizations is long and impressive.

It would be hoped that they would aid us in defining a Physician as opposed to just a doctor, but I do not believe that is happening. Granted, my knowledge of and exposure to the vast majority of these organizations is limited. Most of these organizations have published a code of ethics for their membership. If my experience is typical, once written, the code is posted for the members; they are then exposed to the code only if they inquire or look for it. Most medical organizations have evolved into multifaceted operations that involve promoting their particular field of interest. They publish research in that field, produce educational events, and establish practice guidelines, while allowing for a social structure for their members. They become and maintain a strong political voice at the national level for the interests of the specialty with the National Institutes of Health, Medicare, Congress, and the current government administration.

Medical societies formed by specialists usually begin their development from the association of well-meaning doctors with similar interests. These well-meaning doctors are most commonly from academic medicine. Practicing doctors do not normally have the time, resources, or ability to participate. Ultimately, the academicians organize as a business to recruit additional doctors with a similar interest and to promote that area of interest. The organization grows by adding members. Practicing doctors will make up the majority of the membership, but the academic and organizational doctors will be the major driving force. The organization will establish membership categories, often including one titled "Fellow" of the organization, to denote members with special expertise in that field. The status is achieved by satisfying criteria set up by the organization. As the organization develops, the criteria frequently become less rigid, and in many organizations, the title is given solely based on membership (paying the organization's required yearly dues).

Organizational staff members are added to facilitate the operation and its growth. Awareness of their special interest is needed as well as money for research into the medical problems involved. More staff members are then needed and hired to explore these issues. A director is needed as the doctors do not have the time to do that work. Under the professional administrator, the organization grows and prospers. The administrator and employees work to achieve the original goals, while expanding and growing the organization's influence. A business is born.

Medical organizations go through these steps and become mature businesses. They become bureaucracies unto themselves. A medical organization's survival is like that of any other business. Management must become redirected to some degree to continue to create a need for its existence and pay for its efforts. Almost always, medical societies come into existence to perpetuate a high quality of the work in the specialty they represent. As a business grows, its original goals are given recognition and attention, but for the business to continue, finances become a driving factor. The appearance of the business to the outside world becomes a major area of concern. The same happens with medical organizations. Government agencies must look with favor upon the organization before members can acquire grants to continue their research. The societies become politically active. The business takes on a life of its own. As in all large businesses, the organization's income often becomes the main focus and object of its activities, rather than the original product or purpose which led to its creation.

Around the time I completed my specialty training, the highest accolade a doctor in my field, internal medicine, could achieve was to be selected as a Fellow in the American College of Physicians (ACP). The College required members to show evidence of clinical care and academic excellence to receive the distinction. The latter was defined as having published five medical papers. Several years after my training, I applied for fellowship status when I had only published four papers.

I was turned down for advancement to the status of Fellow. You rightly note that I did not meet the criteria, and I didn't. But my fourth paper was a three-year major series on staging lung cancer. It had taken hundreds of hours of work. For the next several years, that same organization quoted it as a landmark work in the field. But alas, it only counted as one publication. The next year and another couple of publications later, I was made a Fellow. It was the number of publications, not their merit, that had counted.

That experience led me to question what constitutes merit. What makes a doctor a good doctor, a Physician? As the decades passed, my skepticism grew about how we view and assess the quality of medical doctors. After almost forty years as a member of the ACP, I had another interaction with them. I asked about a possible reduction in membership fees because of my senior years, as most societies provide for such a reduction. I was told that it was not possible. In addition, I was informed that, if I did not pay the full amount of my dues, I could not use the title of "Fellow" of the college. The honor of continuing to be called a Fellow in the American College of Physicians is apparently only available by paying a yearly stipend.

Medical organizations, it seems to me, often evolve into working as a business first and then continue operating to grow themselves into a bigger and more important business. They succumb to enlarging their business by thinking "while we are doing this, why don't we add ______?" My experience is admittedly limited, but many medical organizations appear to undergo this process, and seldom do those medical societies or groups represent their primary stated interest above that of their business needs.

In the 1960s, medical specialty board examinations originated in the subspecialty fields of medicine. They were generated by and from the early specialty societies. Once passed, they were a mark of excellence, a marker that one had achieved a high level of proficiency in one's field. Now, over fifty years later, there are specialty boards for almost every field. In most fields, passing a specialty board is a minimum requirement for working in that field. Hospitals, clinics, insurance companies, and other medical organizations will limit one's participation based on board certification. As the number of doctors taking board certification testing grew, the medical organizations created independent businesses to handle the process. These businesses have grown into monopolies that now set the rules.

Board certification is probably one of the clearest examples of a medical organization's efforts to define excellence evolving into a business monopoly. Its stated goals are to define and maintain physician quality, but it appears that its operations are designed to perpetuate and make money for the business at the expense of those physicians. Board certification, once a sign of quality, is now a sign of working in the system. Almost all doctors have them, including the excellent, the average, and the others.

Medical society memberships and board certifications can indicate academic excellence, appropriate associations, and achievements of the member doctors. While important factors describing a doctor's interest, qualifications, and work, they do not distinguish the Physician from the doctor. The Physician should be more than what these represent.

Who, then, Is a Physician?

What does it take to be a Physician? There is no standard to guide us. There are no set goals for a Doctor of Medicine to strive toward to be considered a Physician. The distinction may be one of my own making. I believe it is real because of my fifty years as a medical doctor, with thirty-five of those years practicing medicine alone or in small groups. Medical doctors, like all workers and professionals, vary in their knowledge, personalities, skills, and ethics. Is the distinction important? I think it is and should be recognized by the profession and general population.

As a human engaged in my life's work, I would like to be the best doctor of medicine that I can be. I would like to be able to recognize the standards that define the best of my profession. I would like others to be able to recognize that I have reached those standards. Presently, such standards are not defined, are not recognized, and certainly are not agreed upon.

Recognitions of excellence as a practicing doctor of medicine by anyone but the patient and the doctor are driven by publicity, by academic institution affiliations and titles, as well as by professional societies and standards. All may identify excellent doctors, but most only identify notoriety and intellectual achievements, not what these pages have described as qualities a Physician would exhibit. I have already expressed my views on professional societies and board certifications and their failure to identify Physicians. Public, academic, and economic recognition of doctors should also be considered.

Society and the public note doctors through local publications, advertisements, hospital appointments, and other sources. The politically active, entrepreneurial, self-aggrandizing, and administrative doctors are all more likely to be known. The doctors meeting and seeing patients are not. Yes, there are word-of-mouth recommendations from patient to patient, but those are limited by geography, insurance, and government rules and regulations. Word does not get out of the neighborhood.

Doctors in academic and semi-academic environments are subject to institutional norms and beliefs. Being a Physician for the patient in that environment is difficult, as most patient care, at best, is with one trainee between the doctor and the patient. Often, there are two or three trainees separating the professor or educator from the patient. Success is defined by research and publications, not by patient care.

The financial world of medicine does not recognize quality. Governments and insurance companies see our work as a step in an assembly-line process. In their eyes, while caring for the ill, the best doctor in the world is worth no more that the mediocre. A code for the service provided is the service. That is all the payer sees. One doctor might save a life with a half-hour visit and a simple prescription; the other might order thousands of dollars in testing for the same patient and have no concept of the diagnosis. A doctor whom the patient has searched out to consult might be an authority on the patient's problem, while another may not even recognize the problem. They are paid the same.

Self-recognition that we have reached the pinnacle of our career is actually all we should expect of our time in this world. Like the eldest brother in Thomas Cleary's ancient Chinese legend, whose skill is never known outside his village, I believe Physicians, not doctors, recognize their achievements and need no other rewards to consider their life a success. We are just ourselves, solely what we think and believe we are. Do others recognize those differences in the quality of a doctor's work? Only those looking for a personal Physician actually do so.

What, then, is a good definition of a Physician? I should know, but I don't. A set of values, an Oath, is important, but that alone does not make a Physician. Other qualities are important. The Physician will enjoy the people who are his patients, enjoy learning about them and hearing their stories. A physician expects all types of individuals to pass through his care. Listening and talking with them is an important part of their care. Being able to talk to laborers and college professors alike in a manner that they understand is an important trait. A Physician will not agree with the opinions, lifestyles, and attitudes of many of his patients, but that will not affect his communications with them, recommendations for them, or care of them.

One of my favorite poems is by Sam Walter Foss. It is titled *The House by the Side of the Road*, and it describes the attitude I believe Physicians should maintain with their patients. Here is a portion of that poem.

The House by the Side of the Road

There are hermit souls that live withdrawn
    In the peace of their self-content;
There are souls, like stars, that dwell apart,
    In a fellowless firmament;
There are pioneer souls that blaze their paths

Where highways never ran; –
But let me live by the side of the road
And be a friend to man.
. . .
Let me live in my house by the side of the road
Where the race of men go by –
They are good, they are bad, they are weak, they are strong,
Wise, foolish – so am I.
Then why should I sit in the scorner's seat
Or hurl the cynic's ban? –
Let me live in my house by the side of the road
And be a friend to man.

Yes, a physician should live in a house by the side of the road and be a friend to man.

There is something more, though. It is hard to name. Character is probably the best word to use. To be a Physician, strength of character is required. I am sure there are many Physicians who pass through their careers unstressed and possibly untested. Most do not. There are ethical dilemmas, legal issues, financial disputes, practice conflicts, unhappy patients, and other issues to challenge Physicians as they move through their professional lives. It requires a steadfast awareness of who they are to make the journey, hopefully wiser but undamaged. Another favorite poem of mine describes that strength of character: *If* by Rudyard Kipling.

IF

If you can keep your head when all about you
    Are losing theirs and blaming it on you,
If you can trust yourself when all men doubt you,
    But make allowance for their doubting too;
If you can wait and not be tired by waiting,
    Or being lied about, don't deal in lies,
Or being hated, don't give way to hating,
    And yet don't look too good, nor talk too wise:

If you can dream – and not make dreams your master;
    If you can think – and not make thoughts
    your aim;
If you can meet with Triumph and Disaster
    And treat those two impostors just the same;
If you can bear to hear the truth you've spoken
    Twisted by knaves to make a trap for fools,
Or watch the things you gave your life to, broken,
    And stoop and build 'em up with worn-out tools:

If you can make one heap of all your winnings
    And risk it on one turn of pitch-and-toss,
And lose, and start again at your beginnings
    And never breathe a word about your loss;
If you can force your heart and nerve and sinew
    To serve your turn long after they are gone,
And so hold on when there is nothing in you
    Except the Will which says to them: 'Hold on!'

If you can talk with crowds and keep your virtue,
Or walk with Kings – nor lose the common touch,
If neither foes nor loving friends can hurt you,
If all men count with you, but none too much;
If you can fill the unforgiving minute
With sixty seconds' worth of distance run,
Yours is the Earth and everything that's in it,
And – which is more – you'll be a Man my son!

If the doctor can, the doctor may be a Physician.

Who, then, is a Physician? At best, I have tried to describe the role, but I am not able to define it. I believe it is characterized by the doctor performing their role and interacting with the individuals under their care in an exemplary manner. It is about the care of the individual. A physician's primary role is always focused on the care of the patient. Whether a general practitioner in a rural community or the CEO of a healthcare business, their approach, their perspective, and a Physician's sentiments are focused on the care of the individual. It is a combination of skills that comes with confidence, experience, and knowledge, along with that hard-to-define personality and character.

As a patient, you will know when your doctor is a Physician. It is like Kenneth Clark, a well-known art historian and museum director recognized for his study of civilizations in the last half of the twentieth century, said when asked, "What is civilization?" He responded, "I don't know. I can't define it . . ." But then he added, "I can recognize it when I see it." So too will you recognize when your doctor is a Physician.

If you are a doctor working with patients, at some point you'll understand. You will know. Maybe it is when you are the best you can be at your job. Maybe it will be when, as Joseph Cambell said, you feel your "bliss." You will know when you are a Physician. Enjoy your journey! Few have the opportunity, and even fewer reach the pinnacle of the profession.

Epilogue and a Calling

SECTION FOUR

Epilogue and a Calling

In this book, I have attempted to describe the characteristics of a Physician. As I worked through my thoughts, revised and rewrote these pages, it struck me how the nobility and importance of our work seems to fade from our lives and minds with time. It is diluted by the magnitude of the calling and our limited successes. The irrationality, insensibility, and lack of nobility of many working in healthcare and the business side of medicine contribute to the cloud that appears over our ideals. A reminder of the tradition of our ancient art and its noble goals needs to be part of our principles and work.

A universal oath and pledge day should be recognized by all providing care for the ill. A day when we review our oath or pledge to the noble goals of our profession. On that day we should repeat, read, or recite to ourselves and to others, if possible, the oaths and pledges of our profession. A review once a year would greatly increase their presence in our minds.

July first has been the start of the newly graduated doctors' and advanced providers' entry into the working world of medicine. It is the day I have chosen as my oath day. If the reader is a provider, I would ask that they join me on that day and repeat their oath.

The Hippocratic Oath that follows is not an exact duplicate of the one I took those fifty-seven years ago. That one is lost to time. I have adapted a modification of the Oath presented earlier in this volume. It takes into account the changes in how doctors are trained and the narrowness of the fields of practice that have occurred in medicine over the past two and one-half millenniums.

For completeness, I have included forms of the Nightingale Pledge and the Physician Assistant Oath for use by those providers if they would happen on this book. The reader may not agree with the forms selected for inclusion and may want to use the one they swore to before or modify these, but that is not important. What is important is the annual reaffirming and recognition of our commitment to the higher ideals of our profession directing the care of the ill.

A Classical Hippocratic Oath 2025

I swear by my God and by all those I hold dear, making them witnesses—with homage to the gods of Hippocrates' ancient Greece, Apollo the physician, Asclepius, Hygeia, Panacea, and by all their gods as well as goddesses—to bring the following oath and written covenant to fulfillment, in accordance with my power and my judgment;

To regard him who has taught me this art and profession as equal with my parents, and to give a share both of rules and of lectures, and of all the rest of learning, to my children, to the children of those who have taught me, and to the pupils who have made both a written contract and sworn by a medical convention but by no other.

And I will use regimens for the benefit of the ill in accordance with my ability and my judgment, but from what is to their harm or injustice, I will keep them.

And I will not give a drug that is deadly to anyone if asked for it, nor will I suggest the way to such counsel.

And in a pure and holy way I will guard my life and my art and profession.

I will not cut unless trained to do so, but I will cede those surgeries and special procedures to practitioners trained for those activities.

Into as many houses as I may enter or lives as I may influence, I will go and work for the benefit of the ill, while being far from all voluntary and destructive injustice, especially from sexual acts, both upon women's bodies and upon men's, both of the free and of the slaves.

And about whatever I may see or hear in treatment, or even without treatment, in the lives of human beings—things that should not ever be divulged outside—I will remain silent, holding such things to be unspeakable, sacred, and not to be divulged.

If I render this oath fulfilled and if I do not blur and confound it making it to no effect, may it be granted to me to enjoy the benefits both of life and of my art to be held in good repute among all human beings for time eternal. If, however, I transgress and perjure myself, the opposite of these.

Nightingale Pledge*

I solemnly pledge myself before God and in the presence of this assembly to pass my life in purity and to practice my profession faithfully.

I shall abstain from whatever is deleterious and mischievous, and shall not take or knowingly administer any harmful drug.

I shall do all in my power to maintain and elevate the standard of my profession and will hold in confidence all personal matters committed to my keeping and all family affairs coming to my knowledge in the practice of my calling.

I shall be loyal to my work and devoted towards the welfare of those committed to my care.

*From Farrand Training School Grace for Nurses 1893

Physician Assistant Oath

I solemnly pledge to hold the health, safety, welfare, and dignity of all human beings as my primary responsibility.

I will uphold the ethical principles of patient autonomy, beneficence, nonmaleficence, and justice in all aspects of my practice.

I commit to pursuing lifelong learning and professional growth to ensure the highest standard of care.

I will treat all individuals who seek my care with fairness and compassion, holding in confidence the information entrusted to me in the course of practicing medicine.

I will work collaboratively with my fellow healthcare professionals to provide compassionate and effective care, always striving to contribute my knowledge and experience to the betterment of the community.

With integrity, I will respect the professional relationship between physician assistants and physicians, continuously sharing and expanding knowledge within my profession.

In all that I do, I will remain dedicated to the service of others, honoring the trust placed in me as a physician assistant.

Final Thioughts

In closing, I will share these final thoughts. Several years ago, as I reflected on how I got to that point in my life, I wrote these words. They express the thoughts on my career through its early phases, from my early positions and from before entering medicine as I held numerous odd jobs to pay for my education.

Becoming a Physician

I could have been a laborer if I had not been so inquisitive.

I could have been a builder, but I would have been a better laborer.

I could have been an architect if I had any artistic skill.

I could have been a man of business if it had a higher moral purpose.

I could have been a musician if I had learned the language of music.

I could have been a forest ranger if I had followed my heart.

I could have been a wanderer if I had not met the love of my life.

I could have been a writer if I could spell.

I could have been a soldier doctor if I believed in war.

I would have been a research scientist if I believed "p" values proved something.

I would have been an academic if I believed medicine to be a set science.

I would have been a physiologist if I believed the equal pressure point theory of airflow limitation.

I am a trained doctor, but as a Physician, I am self-taught and mentor-shown.

I am honored to be a member of the ancient band of healers sworn to the Hippocratic Oath as witnessed by my God with respect for Apollo and Asclepius.

I have followed the steps of my mentors to the best of my abilities.

I am a Physician, a husband, and father to my four-legged children. I am happy.

RGH 29406

Bibliography

Most of this book is based on my experiences, readings, and opinions. There are a few resources that are referred to in the text that the reader may want to review.

Thomas Cleary's Chinese legend of the emperor's physician and his family of physicians:

Sun Tzu, Thomas Cleary translator. *The Art of War.* Shambhala Publications Inc. Boston and London. 1991.

There are many articles on the Hippocratic Oath. For an in-depth review, a search of your own is warranted. The two articles below are the source of the Oath used here and provide an excellent starting point.

Helen Askitopoulou and Antonios N. Vgontzas. *The relevance of the Hippocratic Oath to the ethical and moral values of contemporary medicine. Part I: The Hippocratic Oath from antiquity to modern times.* Eur Spine J. 2018 Jul;27(7) 1481-1490.

Helen Askitopoulou and Antonios N. Vgontzas. *The relevance of the Hippocratic Oath to the ethical and moral values of contemporary medicine. Part II: Interpretation of the Hippocratic Oath - today's perspective.* Eur Spine J. 2018 Jul;27(7) 1491-1500.

The excesses and mistakes of doctors are not hidden. Most families have their own stories. For exposure to what ambition and greed will do to some who have received the Doctor of Medicine degree and how far they stray from care of the patient, I would recommend three books. These books on the history of the pharmacological industry, the business takeover of the medical profession, and the business of medical scientific publications highlight some notable and egregious examples of doctor behaviors.

Gerald Posner. *Pharma.* Avid Reader's Press. New York, NY. 2020.

Stanley Wohl. *The Medical Industrial Complex.* Harmony. New York, NY. 1984.

Richard Smith. *The Trouble with Medical Journals.* Royal Society of Medicine Press Ltd. Ashland, Ohio. 2006.

The following book has been in my possession for sixty years. It is a treasure and contains "The Deacon's Masterpiece," "The House by the Side of the Road," and 'If." All three poems are available online from multiples sources.

An Anthology Compiled by Roy J. Cook. *One Hundred and One Famous Poems, with a Prose Supplement (Revised Edition).* The Reilly & Lee Co. Chicago. 1958.

www.ingramcontent.com/pod-product-compliance
Lightning Source LLC
LaVergne TN
LVHW100316210926
848480LV00003B/1139

* 9 7 9 8 9 8 9 3 6 3 1 2 4 *